CW00448936

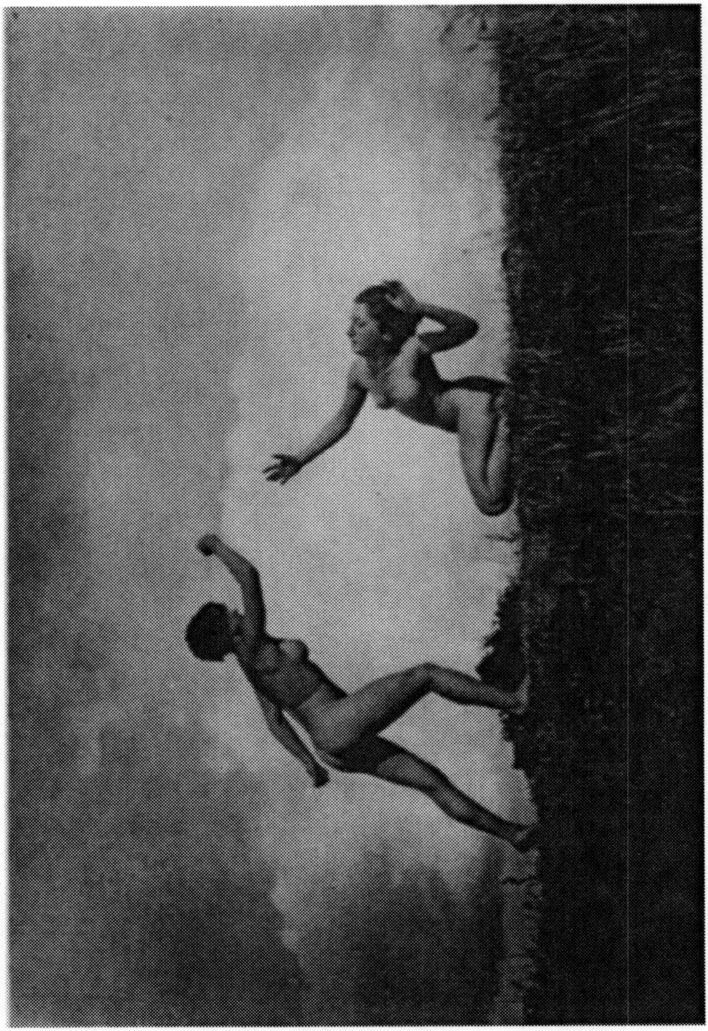

AMONG THE NUDISTS

FRANCES AND MASON
MERRILL

With an Introduction by

JOHN LANGDON-DAVIES

"*Mislike me not for my complexion,*
the shadowed livery of the burnished sun."
MERCHANT OF VENICE, ACT I, SC. I, 2.

1931
LONDON
NOEL DOUGLAS

NOEL DOUGLAS

PROPRIETORS : WILLIAMS AND NORGATE LTD.
38, Great Ormond Street, W.C.I.

PRINTED IN U. S. A.

To

M.-K. DE MONGEOT

and the

AMIS DE VIVRE

We wish to express our gratitude to John T. Flynn for invaluable advice regarding our manuscript, and to Dorothy Pearson and Aline and Lawrence Cramer for assistance and for moral encouragement in facing the disgrace of this scandalous public confession.

For the illustrations, we gladly acknowledge our indebtedness to: Josef Bayer (for the frontispiece and pictures facing pages 26, 110, 146, and 222); Paul Zimmermann (for pictures facing pages 42, 60, 82, 110, and 132); and Vivre, *of Paris (for pictures facing pages 42, 60, 170, and 194).*

FRANCES *and* MASON MERRILL

November 1930
New York City

INTRODUCTION

THE AUTHORS OF THIS BOOK HAVE ASKED ME TO WRITE an introductory note because, they say, a modest publication of mine, *The Future of Nakedness,* was partly responsible for their interest in the subject. It would however be hard to imagine two more different approaches to the same subject; for whereas mine was Utopian and suggested that in the future all reasonable governments would insist, on grounds of public morality and health, on the removal of all clothes; theirs describes how many individuals on these same grounds have forestalled such a decree and have learned the art of enjoying the sun and air unfettered.

One book describing European practices of public nakedness has already been prevented from appearing in America by a semi-official authority and there will be many who will dislike the present book. Clean-minded people are rather rare especially among those who devote themselves to keeping art, literature and life pure; so that authors like these must expect to be attacked. Moreover I can see a criticism of what must almost be called a "cult" of nakedness from many people who prefer to remove their clothes in a nonchalant way, when and where they please, without forming a club to do it.

Now the first class of critic must be left severely alone, since we cannot reply or convert them without taking the trouble to clean out the Augean stables, which they are pleased to call their minds. I can only hope that they will take steps against this book, so that its sales may be pleasantly increased. With the second class of critics I have more sympathy. Temperamentally I agree with them. I like women retaining their own names, if they desire to do so; but I do not like the Lucy Stone league; I have certain patriotic feelings for my native soil and poetry, but I hate patriotic societies; I dispense with clothes whenever I can, but I do not need a secretary and a treasurer to help me. But it is certainly true that in these days of increasing social intolerance and grandmaternalism both public and private, one must protect one's inalienable right to the pursuit of sun, health, and happiness by having a definite place and a selected group to share one's rightful exuberances. Until we can all walk down Fifth Avenue with nothing on but shoes and sunshade, there must be clubs and associations such as those described in this book.

I think the authors are to be congratulated on a certain lack of sentimentality which they have achieved. Those who enjoy nakedness must safeguard themselves against the evil states of mind so often caused by the fact of being a minority in the right. They have succeeded here. I wish they did not talk about "nudism": to me people wish to be nude only when they are ashamed to be naked; but that is a personal reaction to philology.

Introduction

I believe the book as a whole will be valuable especially because it shows the movement towards a greater enjoyment of nakedness as emanating not from cranks, aesthetes, emotionally unstable people such as often try to live entirely on nuts, to discover perpetual motion, and to tell you all about their Oedipus complex, but from athletic, out-door people with plenty of energy and a very few isms. As such it ought to appeal to Americans and we can look forward within a reasonable number of years to summer camps where the pallor of the city will be washed off in the lotion of air and sunbeams. It is not as a means of making the sick healthy, that the reader should consider this book and the facts it describes, but as a means of making the healthy more healthy and happier too.

I notice, especially towards the end of the book, several quotations from my own little brochure. These have suffered a sea change. It would not be true to suggest that I tried to influence people in any way; but were I a proselytiser I should certainly try to *laugh* people out of their clothes. The laughter has been left out by my quoters. This is I think a mark of progress; for in my generation we could only approach the subject through wit, in theirs it is possible to be serious. Reforms often come like that; at first reformers are a little shy of their own reforms, and they introduce them with a laugh; then their followers develop more boldness and the laughter is no longer necessary. This book shows that the fight for nakedness has entered a second stage and it remains for the reader to carry on the battle to a final victory.

JOHN LANGDON-DAVIES

London, 1931

AMONG THE NUDISTS

FOREWORD

A YEAR AGO LAST SUMMER, ON SUNDAY AFTERNOONS, when the sun had reached the south windows of a certain Manhattan apartment, a light-starved young couple used to open the upper half of the windows, screen the lower panes from the view of the Titanic Tower across the way, and take sunbaths in a slender strip of light three feet long and a foot wide. There was no danger of sunburn even if the full intensity of the violet rays could have penetrated the soot-laden atmosphere of New York; in an hour or so, as the sun slipped behind the Titanic Tower to remain concealed in back of the taller buildings to the west, the little band of light would flicker out.

But even New Yorkers have vacations—for two weeks. This couple sought the spot in Maine that seemed farthest removed from railroads and motor highways, from the city evils that are at their worst in New York, the apotheosis of cities. Once or twice on a lonely hilltop, walled in by evergreens through which no trail led, this couple ventured to sunbathe in the open air. In the shelter of the pines, on the good green earth, in the pure atmosphere of the country, they felt the life-giving power of the sun as it had not been possible to feel it in the polluted city air. But the mental relaxation and enjoyment that should accompany physical well-being were imperfect. Fearful, they listened to every sound, watched each stirring of the surrounding trees, and started when a twig snapped in the brush; with tense muscles they were ready at an instant's alarm to snatch their clothes and flee. They were prey to visions of a rural jail.

A year later this same couple was frolicking in sunny glades with a crowd of men, women and children, playing games, doing gymnastics, swimming, or basking in the sun upon the sand—all in the costume and innocence of Eden before the serpent. What is more, their earthly paradise was not a South Sea island untouched by missionaries and their calicoes, nor yet the jungles of darkest Africa. It was in the heart of civilized Europe, and its denizens belonged to the white race, were educated, even cultured, men and women.

Neither was theirs the only one of such paradises. There are many of them. But perhaps most amazing of all to an American is the fact that such assemblies are not surreptitious; their meeting places are known, even advertised. Indeed, some of them are not even walled in, only a wire or a ditch and a "private" sign marking the boundaries. The curious can stray in unhindered—though they do not. And as for the police, it is no affair of theirs. To be sure, not all of these paradises are open to the public: some of them are only for members of a club or league; others can be entered by anyone proving his good faith and character; but all are legal.

Incredible to an Anglo-Saxon? Certainly it would have been so to our New York couple a year ago. But this is the story of their Odyssey.

CONTENTS

AMONG THE NUDISTS

I

NACKTKULTUR ASSAILS US

THE LONG ANTICIPATED REST AND RELAXATION OF A SLOW North Atlantic crossing in early summer had distinctly not been realized. Instead, between an altogether unseasonable arctic atmosphere and days of storm and seasickness, we landed in Germany, the starting point of our long-planned visit to Europe, in anything but the proper physical condition for travelling. And this after we both had worked so hard through the first spring heat to get away! It was disheartening.

But to Herr Koenig, the young German who had received our letters of introduction in Hamburg, our plight was easily remedied. All we needed was rest and—gymnastics.

A vacation spent in doing setting-up exercises scarcely appealed to us, but the idea of rest seemed reasonable. We were thinking vaguely of postponing our tour by a few days, perhaps a week, when he startled us by proposing that we give ourselves two weeks, if not a month. He suggested a place up near the Baltic, a short way from Hamburg, the *Freilicht-park* of Klingberg, where he had just spent his own two weeks' vacation; he could make all the necessary arrangements for us, and the cost would be reasonable.

Certainly his own physical condition was a fine testimonial: clear blue eyes laughed out of a round German face that was burned to a russet brown; his whole being seemed to exude health and vitality. When we asked for a few details about this place so "*wunderbar*," he hastened off—with a haste that at once gave us misgivings—for a big album of snapshots he had taken.

Our hearts sank. While he arranged chairs so as to seat himself between us, we glanced hopelessly at one another with sickly smiles, prepared for at least a half hour's boredom of looking at vacation pictures, in all likelihood so fuzzy and indistinct that they would have to be explained.

He opened the album.

Good God! The first page was taken up by a single photograph—one might well say a full-length portrait—at least 8 x 10, apparently an enlargement, of Herr Koenig himself, leaping high in the air to catch a ball, and—naked as a newborn sparrow!

We, the guests, each heard the other gasp and, without seeing, felt the other blush.

"*Schön, nicht war?*" murmured Herr Koenig rapturously, as usual forgetting his English in his emotion.

Fortunately his comment, though in form an interrogation, called for no reply from us. We were deathly silent.

The effect of that first picture was staggering, stunning. Had we been the least prepared for it, at all forewarned, we could have reacted in some fashion or other; but coming so unexpected, all-at-once and out of the black (of that album), it nearly paralysed us. Never would we have suspected Herr Koenig of exhibitionism.

Happily our friend was too enthralled to notice our confusion. Completely engrossed in the picture, he was for a few moments quite unconscious of even our presence; he was captivated by the sheer beauty of the thing—a beauty quite lost on us, however. This gave us time to recover.

And then, as the pages were turned, came other pictures—hundreds of them, it seemed—but smaller ones, several to the page. All were of nudes, unadorned by so much as a fig leaf, taken in the open air, singly or in groups, of both sexes, all ages, sizes, heights, beautiful and ugly, a whole galaxy of human forms in every conceivable posture and position, in action and repose.

Later we recalled how, when there appeared a picture of an especially beautiful young girl and Herr Koenig would demand, "*Herrlich, nicht war?*" we wondered at his brazen depravity.

So this was the place and the way he would have us go to rest and recuperate! The idea of such a thing was just a bit too fantastic. We felt as we might were someone to say to us, "Come, step into my rocket-ship and we'll go to Mars for tea." It seemed totally unreal to us.

In spite of his arguments and urging, we finally broke away, pleading the need of time in which to make a decision.

Decision! As if that required any time on our part! The whole business was too preposterous to be even considered. We left with mingled emotions of anger and pity, uncertain whether his proposal was an insult or merely a sign of his aberration.

We were barely out of Herr Koenig's house and again on the streets of Hamburg when we were confronted with magazines which, judged from the pictures ornamenting the covers, were devoted to the nude. A few such we had noticed the day before, as soon as we had got off the boat train; but we had then taken them to be a special product for sale to the tourist. With our limited knowledge of the native tongue we had surmised the pornographic appeals subtly implied by the voice of the vendors who, thrusting their wares before our eyes, repeated again and again their "*Schön, nicht war? Sehr schön!*" Now we saw these things as something else, a native product for native consumption, for they seemed to be on sale everywhere.

We had heard not a few people in the past condemn the Germans for being addicted to this sort of thing, for blatant obscenity, views we had always tended to discount as being based more on national prejudice than a knowledge of facts. These magazines, however, seemed a substantiation, for they were not only offered in abundance and in a diversified choice, but openly, without the least fear or even pretended surreption.

What a paradise this for an Anthony Comstock, for the John Sumners, and all of the Society for the Suppression of Vice!

And yet, these cover pages, now that we came to notice them, did have a singular beauty. They seemed to lack the insinuating naughtiness of implication and coquetry that characterize our own pornographic art. In fact, these pictures left nothing whatever to suggestion. They were brutally frank in their display of everything æsthetic and otherwise pertaining to the human animal.

But theirs was a naïve sort of frankness. They were pictures generally of beautiful young men and women at play in woods and fields, of usually less beautiful fathers and mothers with children of various ages, engaged in games or bathing in sunny waters and in the open air. There was something honest and clean about them that attracted us in spite of ourselves; we were inclined to buy one and examine it. Perhaps it would explain our friend's perversion. But we hesitated, half ashamed and afraid that after all it was nothing but obscenity.

Our interest grew as more and more of these publications were proffered us, not only by the news vendors of every street and park but at the news-stand in our own hotel. It was not until we stopped before the window of a large and obviously reputable bookstore in the business centre of the city, and there found a whole collection prominently displayed—at least twelve or fifteen different titles—that our curiosity overcame our scepticism. Furtively we entered and, with simulated casualness, thumbed one or two of them; then, selecting a couple of the least pretentious, we nervously paid the price asked of us, hurriedly rolled them—covers innermost—and fled with them and our guilty consciences.

Back in the seclusion of our hotel, door securely locked, we proceeded to examine our purchases. What we found was not the pornographic feast that we had suspected, but rather a collection of almost amusingly ingenuous pictures of unclothed German children and adults, dancing and in repose, in the most pastoral surroundings, adolescents gambolling in idyllic settings, and whole shoals of human fish stranded and lying scattered on the hot sands of summer shores.

With much thumbing of dictionaries, we proceeded to investigate the generous accompaniment of printed text. Here again we found the same innocent freedom from any sort of innuendo. In fact it had a distinctly moral tone. It was downright and sincere propaganda for nudity, advocated for the healthy as for the ill, as a preventive as well as a cure, and on moral and psychological no less than purely physical grounds. *Nacktkultur* (literally culture of nakedness), the whole German nudist movement and philosophy, was spread before us.

Of course we had heard of nudism abroad, heard tales and read newspaper accounts, but they had been generally the products of exaggerated rumour or the strained imagination of raconteur or of reporters pressed to fill allotted columns of space, stories obviously sprung from either a gossipy taste for the scandalous or a flair for the sensational. Invariably they had dealt with the subject in the most distant and vaguest manner possible. They had depicted some single group, some isolated camp or centre, and treated it as something either unique or a radical instance—an awful example—of the goings-on in some far-off land and of a foreign people, the victims of a warped psychology. Never had we heard of nudism as a movement, or of nudity as a practice based on a rounded philosophy of life.

Here, on the other hand, we found arguments favouring it, presented seriously and documented by citations from seemingly impeccable authorities in the fields of both science and philosophy. Innumerable were the benefits that these articles attributed to nakedness. They stressed the need of the human organism, particularly of the glandular and nervous systems, for sun- and airbaths, and the superiority of exercises taken unclad to sports or gymnastics practised with even the scantiest athletic costumes.

Clothes through the ages, the unhygienic and unæsthetic garments prescribed by fashions, were discussed, with excursions into anthropology and history, to trace the origins of the sense of modesty and shame. From the varying standards of different cultures, the writers demonstrated that nudity was not shameful in some of the greatest periods of mankind—for instance, in the highly civilized era of Greece, or in the deeply religious Middle Ages; in short, that modesty has no connexion with morality.

Total nudity is chaste, they repeated; it is the suggestion of semi-undress that is indecent and harmful. Hence nudity in common, without distinction of age or sex, is innocuous; nay more, they argued, it is morally profitable. Destroying the secrecy and mystery of sex, it does away with unhealthy desires and perversions, and makes easy the task of giving the young a rational attitude towards sexual matters. The race will profit æsthetically as well, for when people must show their bodies in public they cannot remain complacent about defects and deformities that clothes can mask.

The improvement of the race—that was the goal of *Nacktkultur*. It was not a return to barbarism and a state of nature, but the freeing of man from what is baneful in modern life. The ideal was nothing more startling than the old *mens sana in corpore sano.* The means alone were radical. The whole philosophy might be summed up in the phrase of one writer: "Health, beauty, and purity through nudity and light."

We suddenly realized the significance of the name of Herr Koenig's proposed "*Freilichtpark.*" It did not mean a park of free light in the sense of having gratuitous lighting, free gas or electricity; it meant a park in which the open light of day, the sunlight—and incidentally the open air—was free to play upon the human organism. Likewise, the term "*Lichtfreunde,*" so often repeated in all the articles we read, distinguished the friends of this movement for open, or free, light and air.

Herr Koenig's suggestion no longer seemed so monstrous. Impressed with at least the apparent sincerity and high purpose of the apostles of the new creed, if with nothing else in their doctrines, we were half inclined to learn more of their practice, to judge for ourselves the miraculous blessings they promised, and to decide whether they themselves were true prophets or—what seemed more likely—the fanatical followers of false gods. At any rate we were ashamed of what we had thought when Koenig first revealed the "new life" to us, and we blushed at the memory of our blushes.

Humbly and apologetically we went back to him—not as converted sinners, however, but as open-minded agnostics. We would not commit ourselves to stay at this nudist colony—this *Freilichtpark* in the obscure place, Klingberg *bei* Lübeck—but we offered to go have a look at it.

"Good!" Herr Koenig pronounced emphatically. "You

will like it and be very grateful to me for sending you. It is much better than going to a *Kur* place, like Baden Baden, and not nearly so expensive."

"Yes," we agreed doubtfully, "but we're not sure we shall like *Nacktkultur*. It's entirely new to us, you know."

"Of course you will," he insisted. "Everybody does—once he tries it. If all the opponents of *Nacktkultur* could be got into a *Freilichtpark*, undressed, just for a day, by evening there wouldn't be any opponents."

He followed up this extravagant assertion by repeating that we ought to stay there for several weeks.

"Well," we conceded, "we'll agree to stay a week or ten days—that is, provided we can stand it after the first look."

Herr Koenig laughed heartily at the idea of anyone fleeing from such an innocent thing as a nudist park.

KLINGBERG FREILICHTPARK

II

ARRIVAL AT THE LAND OF NAKED MEN

A FEW MINUTES OUT OF HAMBURG AND WE WERE AWARE of being in old Holstein. Gentle low hills of sandy soil covered with surging fields of golden grain, pastures of the most vivid green sprinkled with flowers of brilliant yellow and white and blue, and tiny hamlets, mere huddles at cross-roads, of a few old red-brick houses trimmed in gleaming white and crowned with high pointed roofs of thatch. A pastoral countryside, a beautiful land indeed, in a quiet peaceful way, that should prove a balm to shattered city nerves, American city nerves.

If one could but forget the ordeal ahead!

Three Germans shared our compartment, a woman and two men, of peasant types with the air of burghers. All were healthy, rosy-skinned animals, and strong. Were they nudists?

The buxom *Fräulein* with the wealth of straw-coloured hair wound around her head, who got on at the next station:

was she too bound for the Klingberg *Freilichtpark?* She vaguely resembled the nude feminine rope-jumper gracing the front cover of *Lachendes Leben* which we had seen on display at all the news-stands of Hamburg the day before.

Did we dare appear before such strangers, clad only in light and air? Could we walk bravely, if not calmly, without a weakening of the knees or a burning blush, before these people? Or would all our Anglo-Saxon heritages rise up to overwhelm us and send us slinking away, terrified by guilt and shame? Should we be able to stand erect, as humans built in the image of God, with these people in their modern Garden of Eden? And if we could, would it be only to find their paradise a sham, a pretext for debauchery that would sicken us?

Such thoughts filled our minds as the country-side sped by our window; every perception came to us associated with this one idea.

An hour and twenty minutes brought us to Lübeck, "The City of Golden Towers" and the chief old Hanseatic port on the Baltic, where we changed trains for another thirty minutes' ride to Dorf Gleschendorf, further up the coast.

The country took on a still more rustic, a primitive appearance, was somewhat rougher and more heavily wooded, with dense forests of beech and pine whose branches brushed the windows of the little train. Paved roads gave way to sandy lanes set deen between hedges of hawthorn, that were occasionally bank full of droves of sheep driven by dogs and slow plodding peasants in caps and corduroys. All was idyllic, a perfect setting for the scenes we had found portrayed in the nudist magazines.

But meanwhile dull grey clouds had covered again the sunny morning sky under which he had left Hamburg, and the breeze was cold with the damp of the sea just beyond the low row of hills. We felt still less inclined to lay aside our clothes and gambol on the grassy slopes. We closed the window of our compartment and turned up the collars of our coats.

As the little train came to a stop at the station of Dorf Gleschendorf, we nervously grabbed our bags and left the compartment, glancing furtively along the platform to see if our golden-haired *Fräulein* was likewise getting off—and, to see how many people took notice of our descent and smiled in full knowledge of our destination. We felt self-conscious, guilty, not a little ashamed.

"Ist dis Mister Merrill?"

We turned to shake the hand of Herr Paul Zimmermann, the owner of the *Freilichtpark,* an alert little man with a shaven face and bald head as brown as a hazelnut, and as clean and smooth.

Strangely enough, he was in knickers and jacket; we had half expected—or feared—to find him nude.

Taking our bags and leading the way to his wagonette, he chatted, in a combination of German, French, and an occasional English phrase or word, and immediately much of our fears and nervousness began to vanish. He was friendly and genuinely human, this little nudist, and we felt drawn to him as to a kind soul in an ugly world.

It was a cold twenty minutes' ride from Dorf Gleschendorf station to Klingberg on the high back seat of the wagonette, along winding roads felly deep in sand that showed no track of an auto. The sky now was a leaden hue; the wind across the fields and heath was sharp. Meanwhile we were regaled with animated talk by Herr Zimmermann, who from the seat ahead pointed out and named the woods and hills and old landmarks along the way.

We learned that he had been twenty-five years building his *Freilichtpark,* and that it still was but the rough beginning of what he planned. He happily told us that we should find English spoken at his place—by a Chinese gentleman, Mr. T. M. Wang, of Shanghai, formerly in consular service in America. In fact, we were going to find the *Landhaus* Zimmermann, he assured us, truly an international institution, being patronized by men and women from not only all parts of Germany but Belgium, England, France, Italy, Switzerland, Austria, Hungary, Australia, and the United States.

After a sharp turn the road dipped and bordered a little lake, perhaps two or two and a half miles wide, surrounded by wooded hills. This, the Grosser Pönitzer See, our host informed us, was where his guests swam, and he proudly pointed out on the opposite shore the clump of trees and a pier which were his property.

A mile further along the lake, at the fork in the road, we entered a tree-arched lane and soon found ourselves at the door of the *Landhaus,* a picturesque red-brick dwelling with high moss-covered roof of thatch, set in a terraced garden of flowers and trees and meandering walks. In every direction one saw woods.

Here we met Frau Zimmermann—looking not more than twenty-five—and the three *Fräuleins,* Sigrun, Waldtraut, and Helga, whose ages ranged from fifteen to twenty. The second, their mother proclaimed proudly, spoke English, but she demurred and with a blush and a shake of the head fled into the house.

Inside, we found the table still set and our noon meal—the principal one of the day, as we were to learn—being kept for us.

We were seated at places on either side of Herr Zimmermann. The maid brought in a salad of raw spinach tops and finely sliced radishes and tomatoes with a thin dressing of vegetable oil. We were gingerly helping ourselves to this when in came a dish of boiled potatoes and a huge bowl of steaming stuff, obviously the *pièce de résistance,* which on closer inspection proved to be—O cruel gods!—unmistakably our favourite abomination, Brussels sprouts. Brussels sprouts, swimming around in some kind of greasy juice and sprinkled over with a brown stuff that looked like sawdust!

We exchanged furtive glances and sickly smiles. What ill luck that we, neither of us vegetarian, should be forced immediately to face—and perhaps leave uneaten—a meal of vegetables!

In answer to a timid inquiry, Herr Zimmermann informed us that the regime in his household was entirely meatless. This was almost too much; to be called upon to sacrifice our tastes in food, our eating habits of a lifetime, along with our modesty! But, there was no visible means of escaping now.

However, the salad proved not so bad after all, and we postponed outright revolt—incidentally committing ourselves, perforce, to helpings from the chief concoction.

Shutting our eyes, we made a valiant effort to squelch our long-rooted revulsion for Brussels sprouts and conveyed meagre forkfuls to our mouths, feeling as must have Socrates when he drank his hemlock. But, strange to relate, the taste in no way resembled the smell of Brussels sprouts.

The juice of this dish we discovered to be a delicious blending of butter and vegetable oils, made extremely palatable by exactly the proper seasoning; and the sawdust that adorned the top turned out to be finely grated nuts. In time we even helped ourselves again—sheepishly, as we caught each other's glance of amused surprise.

Decidedly this non-meat repast was not the hardship we had feared, especially when it was topped off with an excellent Bavarian cream for desert. The only rub was the total absence of anything whatever to wash it down. Not even a glass of water to drink, though this was a shortcoming, we were to find, that was not characteristic of the other two meals of the day, for at breakfast one could have coffee, and at the evening meal a choice of tea, genuine buttermilk, or even "cow-warm" milk.

We came to learn that Zimmermann's was in fact not a strictly vegetarian table, or at least not ruled by any fanatical adherence to such a creed. While following the dietary principle of vegetarianism, the fare was regularly augmented by cheeses at the evening meal, and from time to time even by eggs.

The repast over, we proceeded to the necessary business details with Herr Zimmermann, as Mr. Wang, the English-speaking Oriental, had since come in to act as our interpreter. Through his boyish good offices we first became acquainted with the rules of the *Freilichtpark.*

We found that the privileges of the park were granted only to those seriously interested in *Nacktkultur,* that the burden of proving one's good faith lay wholly upon the guest himself, and that these privileges might even be revoked at any time without Herr Zimmermann being obliged to explain the reason.

The printed rules specified when and where clothes were obligatory—as, for instance, in the *Landhaus* Zimmermann and on the public road between the park and the lake. But in the park itself they might or might not be worn, according to one's choice in the matter, provided that when dressed one did not loiter near the playgrounds or other places frequented by the unclothed, nor in the vicinity of the bathing beach at the lake, where even bathing suits were forbidden. Clothing was to be hung only at designated places. Wine, beer, all spirits, and tobacco were prohibited inside the park limits. And there were several minor regulations.

These read and explained to us, we were each given a blank, formal application for admission. Besides the usual information regarding name, address, age, profession, etc., this called for answers to the following questions:

Are you a member of any organization that is interested in physical culture? What is it called? Where is it situated?

How long have you been acquainted with the Light Movement (Nudism)? How and through whom did you first learn of it?

Are you familiar with the literature of the Light Movement? What books have you read on the subject? What periodicals? Which books and what periodicals do you consider the most valuable?

Have you ever practised *Freikörperkultur* (Free Physical Culture)? Where? Alone or in company with others?

Do you engage in sports? Which ones? Since when? In gymnastics? Which system? Do you swim?

Have you any bodily ailments? What are they?

Somehow the great number and minuteness, even pettiness, of these questions did not strike us as being at all funny. Perhaps it was that our senses of humour had deserted us, impressed as we were by the gravity of our positions, terrified by the ordeal we were facing, and sobered by the whole business of our being there. We now recall only that to us the formality seemed very appropriate to the occasion; we were even gratified at the rigorousness of the regulations.

The catechism finished, we signed our names with all the solemnity of signing certificates of death. That done, we at once set out for an inspection of the *Freilichtpark*, accompanied by Herr Zimmermann and Mr. Wang, with the principal idea of choosing as our abode—for a week or ten days perhaps—either one of the several cabins in the woods or a room in the *Landhaus* Zimmermann, where in either case of course we should board.

Outside the door we found a thermometer registering 13 degrees Centigrade (56° Fahrenheit); a breeze from over the hill struck our cheeks, we thought about divesting ourselves of our clothing and instinctively turned up the collars of our coats. Our guides, bareheaded, sockless, and in sandals, were dressed in two-piece "training suits" of blue jersey, gathered at ankles and waist by elastic bands and open at the throat. In these costumes they looked like a pair of convicts, especially Zimmermann with his hairless head.

Fifty yards up the hill, along a hedge-lined lane, we came to a tight board gate marked "*Privatweg.*" Through it we crossed a small field, where over the treetops we had an excellent view of the lake a quarter of a mile away. Beyond the field, on the first tree of the woodland, we found a sign:

LUFTBADEGELÄNDE
FREILICHTPARK

Zutritt nur mit meiner persönlichen Erlaubnis gestattet. Zimmermann.

[AIR BATH FIELD
FREE LIGHT PARK

Entrance permitted only with my personal authorization. Zimmermann.]

Passing it, we entered the woods and were in the nudist park.

Still no naked men or women adorning the landscape! But when we stopped and listened to the wind sighing through the pines above our heads, and when we glanced up at the forbidding autumnal sky, we thought we understood. No day, this, for sunbathing, and we could scarcely conceive of forgoing our own full quota of clothes.

Thirty feet inside the fringe of trees, in a little clearing, we came to the main field- or park-house. Besides a number of lockerlike dressing rooms, opening outward instead of in —tiny cubical affairs barely large enough to turn around in, with hooks on which to hang one's clothes—this building contained two small rooms downstairs and a larger one above, with beds enough to hold a dozen men.

Through the dense woods of spruce and beech and fir and pine radiated paths of thick sand, soft and smooth, and mossy little trails carpeted with dry needles and dead leaves, with here and there a fallen cone. Despite the chill wind and cheerless day, countless birds sang in the trees, and the air was sweet with the smell of damp earth and growing things. Truly this would be a paradise with sun!

"Guten Tag! Guten Tag!"

Startled, we looked up in the direction of the voice, to the top of the bank above our heads. There, outlined against the grey sky and dark green edge of trees, stood Adam, with body red as a fresh-boiled shrimp.

A man of possibly forty-five or fifty, considerably enlarged about the girth as from having drunk much beer, Herr Krieger, with round gold spectacles and shaven head, answered completely to a certain German type. With the same stiff dignity as if in full attire, he descended the bank to bow above our hands and mutter German welcomes to the Americans.

We, on our part, were not at ease. Suddenly conscious, as never before, of our clothes, we blushed with embarrassment before this man. We felt a positive sense of shame, of impropriety—not on his part, however, but our own. We felt rather as we might on finding ourselves in full evening dress at a social gathering of men and women in sport clothes.

Somehow or other this man completely nude, standing before us so composed, arms folded across his chest, seemed appropriately accoutred, while we, wearing all the clothing we could muster from our summer travelling wardrobe, seemed shockingly misclad. We felt an urge to apologize for appearing as we were. After a painful silence that seemed interminable, we finally mastered our embarrassment and forced ourselves to speak, to make conversation.

In reply to our pidgin German, Herr Krieger assured us that the day was not cold—and strangely there was no slightest sign on his part of chattering teeth, shivering knees, or "goose flesh" along his rosy ribs to belie his words.

Only, he added, one must keep on the move, must run, do "*Gymnastik*" or work—by which, we were to find, he meant cut underbrush, shovel sand, or wheel it by barrow to some of the many new paths and clearings or playgrounds that were constantly being added in the woods. For such work was considered as play by the regular guests of the *Freilichtpark*.

Continuing on around the knoll, we heard the slow beat of a tom-tom in the woods ahead of us, and on a sandy clearing we discovered through the trees two Eves practising a rhythmic dance. Neither of them seemed the least abashed at our approach, this rather fat dull scholar type, the Frau Doktorin Schmiedemann, nor Fräulein Voight, the professional teacher of the dance. Both advanced quite unconcernedly to shake our hands, composed and comfortable, without apparent consciousness of their nudity. Their ease was in striking contrast to our lack of it.

As for us, the moment was excruciating. We knew neither what to say nor where to look. At the same time we felt angry and disgusted with our own self-consciousness. Why should fright and embarrassment so overcome us, make us so abject in the presence of these women without clothes? Fortunately the situation was not prolonged, for after a few words with our host and another shake of our hands, they returned to their dance, leaving us standing on the border of the woods. We steeled ourselves to look at them, to watch them—tight mouthed, perhaps, but without flinching.

To the slow beat of Fräulein Voight's tom-tom they circled, serpentined, now bent forward and now back, their slightly tanned bodies silhouetted sharply against the black background of pines; their arms slowly rising, falling, in unison with their time, mere prolongations of the curving lines of backs and lower limbs.

Suddenly Mr. Wang, excusing himself with the same punctiliousness as if in a salon, dashed off down the path. Returning a moment later, he too was completely nude. Past us into the clearing he bounded, to take a place in the moving tableau. Beside the light skins of the two women, his lithe dark brown body offered a striking contrast as he executed a kind of counter-point to their harmony of motion.

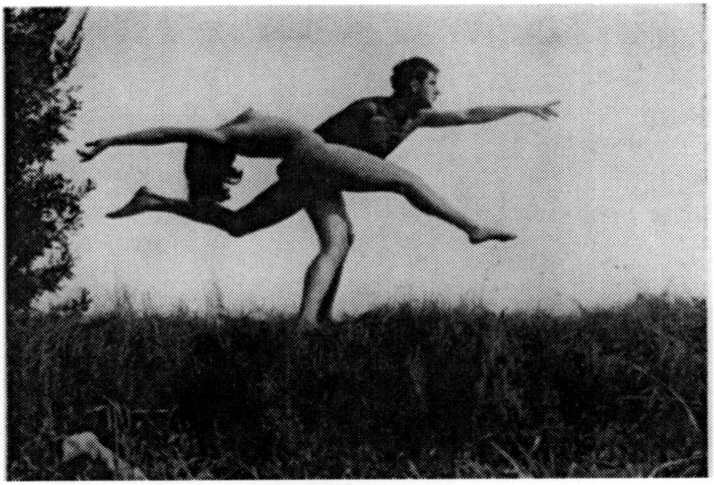

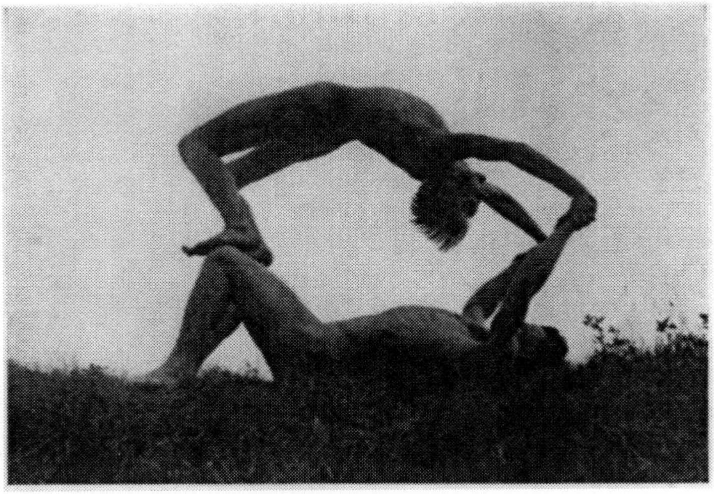

Swaying this way and that, twisting, weaving, their curving bodies and limbs now forming living question marks, now figure O's, the three forms—two light, one dark brown—balanced and paused and glided across the deep green of the woods; their movement was like that of smooth-flowing seagrass in a gently ebbing tide. Despite the ungraceful figure of the *Frau Doktorin,* the trio made a silent symphony there in the otherwise dismal day. We forgot the fact that they were nude, forgot our own embarrassment at watching them; we remained rooted to the spot, silent and lost to ourselves in sheer admiration of the beauty of the scene.

The silence at length was broken by Herr Zimmermann, and we continued our course along the winding paths, circling and traversing the hundred-odd acres of woodland. We inspected the half dozen or so cabins, or *Hütte,* each accommodating two guests; the four or five levelled clearings designed for games or exercises; the sand pit surrounded on three sides by high banks and trees, for quiet baths in the air and sun; the *Moorteich,* or moor pond, fringed with bullrushes and cattails, with a springboard extending out over the deep central pool; and the open-air shower.

Finally, we left the park by a steep path down the hill, crossed the public highway, and visited the lake, where a couple of hardy Eves, just emerged from the forbidding grey waters, were running and shaking and rubbing themselves dry in disdain of towels.

Here we found two more cottages ready for occupancy. But the chill air had already decided us to forgo the seclusion of woodland or lakeside hut for the more comfortable quarters in the *Landhaus* Zimmermann, at least for the present.

Dinner that night, served at a big table that seated Herr Zimmermann and a dozen guests, was another surprise to us. In the centre, on a platter two feet wide, was a kind of layer cake of escalloped eggs and potatoes, garnished with sliced tomatoes and pickles, and the whole sprinkled over with onions chopped very fine. Time after time this platter came around, each guest helping himself generously—for the German appetite, tremendous under normal conditions, when whetted by *Nacktkultur* can scarcely be assuaged. Then really fine butter, and bread—the latter in three grades of brownness—*Schmierkäse,* and a local Holstein cheese, with a choice of tea or fresh milk as beverage. Meat would indeed have been superfluous here.

The evening meals, our subsequent experience demonstrated, were always satisfying, even to confirmed meat eaters. It was harder to accustom ourselves to the noon meal, and more than once we left the table longing for a juicy steak or a browned chop—a craving we later learned how to satisfy.

Supper over, all of us repaired to chairs in an adjoining room, by a hot fire in a big white porcelain stove that nearly reached the ceiling. There, between lusty German songs, which were accompanied by the piano and joined in by everyone but us, Herr Zimmermann, in a spirit most becoming a host, regaled his guests by reciting old folk-tales and whole pages of Nietzsche and Goethe from memory. These he interspersed with interpretative comments, which were listened to with the gravest attention by all who could understand.

At nine thirty, as if in answer to some unquestionable law, everyone arose, again shook hands all around, and with several variations of "Good Night" and "Good Slumber," trooped off to bed. We, the new guests, were shown to a large room under the wide thatched eves, looking out upon the garden, where in a feather bed and beneath a feather comforter we went to sleep, to dream of being discovered nude and chased and stoned through city streets, and of suddenly finding ourselves in our offices back in New York without our clothes.

III

INITIATION

WARM SUN AND THE SONG OF INNUMERABLE BIRDS awoke us in the morning. Somewhere a cuckoo clock was striking, faintly as in another part of the house: "Cuckoo! Cuckoo! Cuckoo!" . . . three, four, five strokes, . . . eight, nine, . . . twelve, thirteen . . . Startled, we looked at our watches, to find the hour seven o'clock.

We rushed to our window only to locate the sound as coming from deep in the forest. After twenty strokes or so it was silent, whereupon an answering note began from the woods of the opposite hill.

Actual cuckoos! Calling to one another with this monotonous regularity, this unbelievably mechanical song! Never again would we doubt the realism of the striking cuckoo clock.

The sun was already high in a sky of the clearest blue. The air, laden with the scent of flowers and pines, was soft with the breath of summer and the nearby Baltic Sea. We dressed hurriedly to go down for a round or two in the garden, to marvel at the variety of flowers there: poppies the size of saucers, making deep splashes of red among the blue and white spikes of giant larkspur; superb big golden globe-flowers, standing erect and proud; spectacular clumps of peonies; whole beds of coquettish pansies; delicate nasturtiums; a fragrant violet-like flower—though larger than any violet ever seen in a florist's shop—and countless others, as well as blossoming shrubs, many we had never known before. Each held a crystal bead of morning dew, and all were the plunder of a million humming bees.

We were astonished at finding no one else enjoying this gorgeous hour. We recalled that on coming through the house we had not seen even a maid in the dining-room. Could it be that all these *Lichtfreunde* were still sleeping, after having retired the night before at ten?

But soon we heard the approach of voices and met Mr. Wang, the *Frau Doktorin,* and half a dozen others coming along the path that led from the *Freilichtpark.* Some were in bathrobes or dressing gowns, some in training suits, some only in trousers and shirts—generously opened at the chest—or light one-piece frocks; all were stockingless, and most of them wore sandals. They informed us that as usual they had arisen, some at six, some at five, some even at sunrise at four o'clock, and were on their way back for breakfast after their customary hour of morning exercise.

But, why had we not been instructed regarding this morning gymnastic schedule? Oh, well, gymnastics were not obligatory for anyone, and all had assumed, as doubtless had Herr Zimmermann, that at least on our first morning we should prefer to sleep. But the next morning? Yes, to be sure, we were welcome to join them if we chose. And it was great fun, they assured us.

Back in the house, we now found the table laid for breakfast. We sat down to a repast that consisted of a dry mixture of uncooked rolled oats, puffed rice, cornflakes, and raisins, eaten barely moistened with fresh milk and sweetened with fruit jelly or marmalade. Again three grades of whole wheat and rye breads, with a big bowl of hazelnuts, and hot coffee to finish off.

The meal over, the park was the order of the day. A few repaired first to their respective rooms, reappearing shortly armed with bath towels, and several of them carrying mysterious little draw-string cloth bags. All started off together, walking and talking, in pairs, in trios, in quartets—all except us. We were too preoccupied to be able to converse with anyone, too wholly absorbed with thoughts of what we were facing. Doubtless we appeared in the eyes of those people as not wanting or needing any company or friends; they probably saw us at that moment as very distant and quite unsociable.

On the way to the park we instinctively lagged behind until we brought up the rear of the little band. We glanced at one another, caught each other's eyes, and nervously laughed; without saying a word, each knew the other's thoughts.

How were we going to stand the forthcoming test? Was our courage sufficient to carry us through the first ordeal, that of undressing before all these strange men and women? We were distinctly conscious of the contrast between our own and their peace of mind, and we were puzzled by it.

Were we abnormally timid, or were they brazen, debased?

We reached the park-house in time to see the first arrivals, stripped of their clothing, trot off up the path into the woods; others were hanging their bathrobes in the locker-like dressing rooms, all the doors of which were standing wide open.

Before us a twenty-year-old *Fräulein,* skirt dropped to the ground about her feet, was pulling a sweater, her only other garment, off over her head; on the terrace above, a young man of twenty-four, her fiancé, completely nude, turned cartwheels while he waited for her to finish. Sitting on the bank, a matronly woman of perhaps forty, one foot raised across the other knee, was concentrating all her attention on the obstinate knot of a shoe string that alone prevented her from being as unclothed as the moment she was born.

So, the locker-like dressing rooms were, after all, merely lockers; the sunny clearing before their doors was the real dressing room!

Unfortunately—or fortunately—we were not attired in a manner to permit any such fireman-like speed of dressing and undressing; we were wearing far too many pieces of clothing, and too complicated, for that. In fact we had scarcely begun the process when the last of the other guests finished and galloped off into the woods, calling back to us to hurry and then come to the game ground in the pines at the top of the knoll.

We hurried.

We took off coats and neckties, carefully hanging them on nails in the least pre-empted locker. We sat down and, fumbling with garters and shoe strings, finally bared our feet. Stepping out upon the damp sand that was still in the shade of the park-house, we shivered, and flinched as if from pain.

With a glance all around, Frances pulled off her blouse, while Mason, in the act of stepping out of his trousers, hastily retrieved them and started at an imagined sound. Both laughed just a bit hysterically, and Frances stepped into a locker and partially closed the door to remove her slip. Mason, left without her moral support, forlornly stood outside unbuttoning—and nervously rebuttoning—his B.V.D.'s. Waiting for her, he told himself.

At this moment a hail came from the direction of the highway, and another guest arrived. Mason reddened, half in his own self-consciousness and half in anger at this breach of their privacy. But without noticing the scowl, the new guest, a man in his early thirties, began sputtering German while he kicked off his sandals and dressing gown. Mason quit rebuttoning his underwear.

"Hurry up, Fran, for heaven's sake!" he called in a tone of irritation.

Turning, he found her cowering in a corner of the locker, undressed down to her undershirt which, with straps already off her shoulders, she still desperately held up. The German, getting no response to his conversation—we hope he attributed it to our non-understanding—stepped forth unclad, a handsome brown figure that soon disappeared up the path into the woods.

Alone again, we silently frowned at each other a moment and then smiled mirthlessly. We resolved to take the plunge, willy-nilly; and hastily, almost recklessly, stripping off chemise and underclothes, we stepped forth out of the shadow of the park-house into the warmth of the sun.

Timidly we started, hand in hand, across the clearing. The sun fell warm upon our backs, and the light touch of the breeze upon our bare skins sent a delicious tingling along our spines. It was as soothing as a warm bath when the body is numb with cold, but invigorating as the shock of a cold plunge when one is hot. We were immediately stimulated, our beings vitalized; our bodies seemed suddenly light and filled with a new strength and a new energy; we felt capable of running with unheard-of swiftness and of leaping very high and far into the air.

From the sunny clearing we entered the cool shade of a wooded path. Our bare feet felt the damp carpet of pine needles and we were suddenly aware to an entirely new degree of all the woodsy smell of the wet morning forest. We were impelled to breathe the air deep down into our lungs, to fill our beings with it and cleanse them. We were intoxicated with an entirely new and utter joy of being alive. We looked at our white bodies and limbs there in the dusky light of the forest, forgot our recent fears and shame, and wanted to run and leap and shout and laugh with our excess of happiness.

Enveloped by the cool damp air, we shivered delightfully and began to trot along our winding wood path, unaware and disdainful of where it led. Low hanging branches showered us with dewdrops of the night before, at the chill shock of which we cried out exultantly and broke into a run. As we raced, twigs of fir whipped our chests and arms, and when a bramble that grazed our thighs caught at the white flesh, the smart was like the thrill of an electric shock.

Suddenly we brought up at the margin of a clearing, the playground where all the guests had come. We had forgotten that we were not alone in the park. Our embarrassment returned; we remembered that we were naked, and, like our first parents, we were afraid. But it was too late to flee; Mr. Wang had seen us.

Abandoning his game he came over to welcome us. At once on our guard, we scrutinized his smiling countenance but found it guileless, innocent alike of all ribaldry and scorn; he was openly friendly, and that was all we could discern.

Yet we did find in his look a candid and obvious curiosity. He frankly took us in from head to feet, while we blushed, shifted our weights nervously from one foot to another, and felt at a great loss for pockets into which to put our hands. We were uncomfortable, but no more than that. For in his eyes there was but that look of those who meet you eye to eye, as if interested and therefore appraising you—something often no more trying than flattering. The next moment he bade us join the games, to which we gladly acquiesced, secretly hoping that our prowess would prove sufficient to distract further attention from our physiques.

Nearly a score of men and women, young and old, were gathered on the playground. One group of six or eight was passing a heavy medicine ball; another was throwing a volley ball about; two pairs were armed with short wooden swords with which they tossed into the air and caught wooden rings about a foot in diameter. Half a dozen other people were merely looking on, or coaching those at play.

Few even noticed us, and they but to smile—friendly smiles—nod, and then turn again to play. Their indifference alleviated our embarrassment. Only the paleness of our skins, in contrast to the pinks and reds and browns of theirs, made us feel conspicuous. Somehow they seemed less nude than we, more naturally and appropriately clothed, and fitting more harmoniously into the setting.

Wang proposed to introduce us to the new game of *Schwingball,* or swing ball, that had just come out, and leading us across the clearing he picked up a contraption that consisted of an inflated leather ball, like a small-sized punching bag, hung from the centre of a ten-foot elastic cord. On either end of this cord was a short wooden stick, equipped with a strap to go around the wrist.

Drawing on the ground with his toe a huge figure "H," perhaps six feet wide by twelve in length—the court in which we were to play—Wang placed one of us in either end and gave us each a stick-end of the cord, so that the ball hung suspended between us, a few inches above the central line of our court. The trick was to keep it swinging there, in a horizontal circle above the ground, while each strove to make it hit the other.

Simple, it sounded, too simple to be highly interesting; but we found it otherwise in fact. Also we were soon surprised to find the degree of genuine exercise it gave; it worked, and worked strenuously, not only the arms—which quickly grew fatigued—but legs and every muscle of the anatomy. And as a game, it proved spectacular, once we had surrendered it to Wang and a German youth who knew its possibilities. Their charges and counter-charges had all the brilliance of a fencing match, plus a great deal more agile play, as first they leaped into the air to let the ball swing under them, and then they crouched—all but flattening themselves upon the earth—so that it would pass above their heads without their sacrificing any ground. It was a contest, a veritable sporting match, as they played it.

But we soon tired of such a strenuous exercise, and joined a dozen other guests who were bound for another clearing in the woods. There they proposed to play what they called "hunter and hare," a game in which the "hunter," outside a thirty-foot ring, is charged with throwing a light volley ball and hitting the "hares" within, whereupon they, as struck, must join with him in trying to hit those still inside the ring.

Such a game, especially when played in the *Lichtkleid* (clothes of light), or park costume, is a favourite one because it calls for much running and jumping in the sun and open air. Nor is it too strenuous—not until you are the "hunter" or "it." Then, alone on the outside of the ring, it becomes extremely difficult to hit the "hares" within, who can easily keep on the opposite side; and every miss on your part calls for retrieving your own wild throws of the volley ball.

This is exciting. One runs and shouts; there is a constant need to "keep the eye on the ball." In the heat of the game we became completely forgetful of ourselves. Hard pounding hearts and heaving lungs are not conducive to self-consciousness.

But a half hour of this and we, the newcomers with muscles still weak, felt justified in quitting for a rest and sunbath in the pit of sand. Secretly, too, we each wanted—and instinctively knew that the other one wanted as well—to be by ourselves for a little while, to confide in one another our first impressions and reactions to this wholly new experience of ours.

This secret hope, however, was not to be realized; we were not the first that morning to seek the sand pit. Half a dozen men and women were already there, stretched out in every conceivable position on the hot white sand. Some, flat on their backs, eyes shut against the sun, had their legs and arms wide spread to gather the full strength of the ultraviolet rays; others were on their bellies to expose their spines to the blistering light.

Most of them were apparently asleep when we arrived, but not so the *Frau Doktorin*, who called to us. We approached almost in fear and trembling, deeply concerned by the grave professional air with which she surveyed our bodies. What, we wondered, did she find wrong with us?

Picking up one of those mysterious little cloth bags that had so aroused our curiosity that morning, she came up the bank. There, crouching on her heels, she pulled it open and turned it upside down. As comb, soapbox, and handkerchief came tumbling out, we saw how nudists solved the pocket problem which had been troubling us. Last came a little bottle of faintly sweet smelling oil, with which she rose and began anointing us.

It was a special preparation for the *Lichtfreunde*, she declared; rather than bleach the skin, it hastened tan, but it prevented blisters, pain, and peeling. What a divinely inspired invention for these modern Adams and Eves!

Our bodies oiled until they gleamed, we stepped down into the pit of blinding white, to find the blistering sand almost unbearable even to our feet. Again the *Frau Doktorin* proved our guardian. Before lying down we had first to kick up a couch of moister and cooler sand from beneath the surface.

Then, flat on our backs, eyes shielded from the sun by our hands, we looked up into the bluest sky we had ever seen, a blue relieved only here and there, down near the surrounding horizon of trees, by small cottony summer clouds.

As we lay there in the quiet heat, all our senses seemed to become more fully awake: we were more keenly aware of the song of birds in the surrounding woods, of the bark of a dog on some distant farm, the whistle of a train somewhere far away, and the thousand summer smells of forest and field.

But shortly it seemed as though the hot sun's rays began to penetrate our skin and, as if by expanding, to relieve the tension of our every muscle and bone. We felt ourselves involuntarily relax, to a degree and in a manner never known to us before. Our bodies seemed to lose all of their rigidity, to be flattening and spreading out with the soft litheness of a cat's.

Peeking through the slits of our fingers, we fell to watching a couple of tiny specks in the limitless blue above. At length they resolved themselves into a pair of vultures, or eagles possibly, floating and soaring in wide slow circles, in lazy effortless circles, by movements which in some strange way came to identify themselves in our minds with the drowsy hum of the countless bees in the shrubs that enclosed the pit, and with the intermittent but monotonous croaking of a bull frog in the *Moorteich* below the hill. A pleasing kind of self-hypnosis came over us and, without quite going to sleep, we sank into a state of semi-slumber filled with sweet dreams and rest.

It was some time later when we were awakened abruptly from this pleasant state by shouts and the appearance on the bank above our heads of some eight or ten persons, of both sexes, fresh from the games. They proposed a swim in the lake before dinner, and they were recruiting their party. Reluctant to bestir ourselves and shake off this pleasing lethargy, we at length succumbed to the temptation of cool waters and agreed to accompany them.

To reach the Grosser Pönitzer See, as we had learned from Herr Zimmermann's regulations, one must put on some kind of clothes, be it nothing more than a bathing suit or a dressing gown, because the trip calls for leaving the borders of the *Freilichtpark* and crossing the public road. And it was here that we came to realize the misfortune of our mode of dress.

In spite of radical curtailments of such utterly superfluous garments as stockings, collars, ties, and vests, we found ourselves woefully encumbered. Barely had we started dressing when the others had on their training suits, their dressing gowns or bath robes, their skirts and sweaters or trousers and shirts, and were on their way to the lake, leaving us to follow them.

After all had gone, there were several minutes of silence

before Mason asked, "Well, what do you think of it?"

"Why, I like it," admitted Frances without a moment's pause. "And you?"

But without waiting for an answer, she continued, enthusiastically, "It's loads of fun, I think; I wouldn't have missed it for anything."

"And all your doubts and hesitations, are they gone?"

"That's the funny part of it to me," she smiled with amusement at the memory. "It all seems so dead easy now and perfectly natural. I was scared to death to begin with; I didn't let you know half how scared I was. When we got out there with all those people, I thought I'd faint if anyone looked at me."

"I must say you concealed it pretty well."

"Oh, as soon as I dared look around enough to see that nobody was paying any attention to us, I got over it. And you, Mick, weren't you scared at all?"

"It took a little nerve for the first minute or two."

"Nothing more than that?" she urged.

"No, really," he insisted. "It was like diving into cold water—hard to start, but all right once you get in. It strikes me this little experience pretty well proves that modesty is an acquired virtue, and not altogether a natural one. If it were innate, you wouldn't get rid of it so quickly and easily."

"And the other people, Mick? Did they shock you any?"

"Not a bit, today, from the moment I got my own clothes off. You weren't shocked, were you?"

"No," she said, and after a moment added, "except a little at myself for not being shocked at such a strange sight."

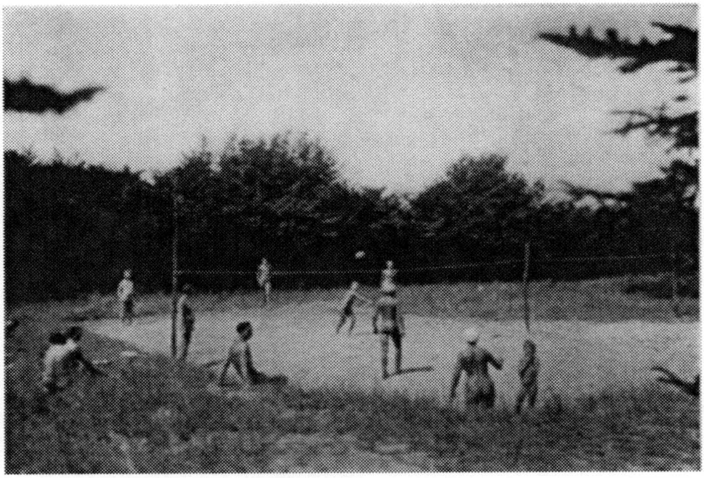

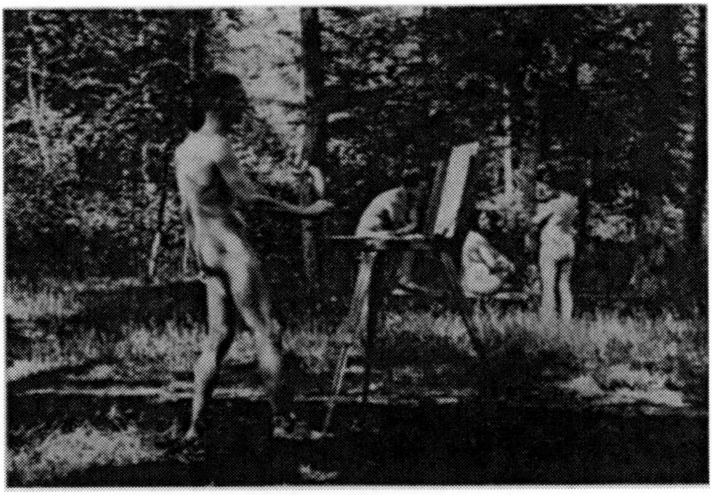

"It's funny, isn't it," he reflected, "how soon you get over all curiosity, and how blasé you get to nakedness? Why, after the first couple minutes, I swear I wasn't interested a bit more in the women than in the men—and I must say I'm not used to being surrounded by naked ladies."

"To tell the truth," Frances remarked, "ever since we set out on this expedition, I've had a sneaking suspicion that we were a little out of our minds. From the moment we told Koenig in Hamburg that we'd try it, I've had a feeling that something was wrong with us for so much as considering such a thing. But now I'm beginning to think we're sane after all. This whole business seems so natural."

"A sure sign of insanity," he grinned. "But frankly, I'm rather sold on it myself. Honestly, I feel like a new man already; a few days of this sort of thing and I'd be all set to go take Italy away from Mussolini. But, aren't you about ready?"

"Ready? For Mussolini?"

"No, dressed, I mean. Come now," he protested, "you don't need that slip thing. Wad it up and I'll stick it in my pocket.

"There's nothing very radical about this business of sun-baths and ultra-violet rays anyway," he pursued as he stowed away the useless garment. "Good Lord, some of our best people at home are religiously doing it because their conservative old family doctor has told them to. And look at the fad last year for sun-back bathing suits; if they're really beneficial, then no suit at all is far . . ."

"You certainly are sold, Mick."

"But seriously, Fran," he countered in a tone of slight embarrassment, "about the only essentially new feature to this movement over here, as I understand it, is that the benefits of sun and air are being sought by relatively hale and hearty human beings, rather than just those with one foot already in the grave."

"That, and this business of having the two sexes take their baths together, indiscriminately," she interrupted.

"Well, as to that too I'm open-minded," he replied, picking up the towels. "I'm thoroughly convinced of the sincerity of these men's arguments about the psychological advantages of nudity in common. Maybe they're mistaken about it, but at any rate they're honest."

"Yes," she agreed with conviction, "and obviously there's something wrong with our prevailing system of sex education. I think it's worth seeing how this system works anyway. We really can't tell much about it in such a short time."

"We haven't noticed any signs of debauchery yet," Mason concluded, as they left the park. "And as for our trying this thing, I don't see how it can possibly hurt us."

IV

THE BEACH WITHOUT BATHING SUITS

FROM THE FREILICHTPARK THE PATH TO THE LAKE plunges down the hill. At first sunless, hewn through a sombre growth of pines, it leaves the limits of the park itself and angles across a sunny clearing and orchard, to emerge in the rear garden of the Waldschänke (Forest Tavern), the hundred-year-old timbered-brick inn that stands at the fork in the road.

The high gabled end of the Waldschänke is crowned by a stork's nest, and about the squat dormer windows of the attic the wide-eaved, mossy, thatched roof sags in soft curves like a sunbonnet out of starch about the face of an old peasant. Quaint and mellow, the tavern fits into its setting, harmonizes with the dark forest of Kronshörn, the big state-owned beech wood across the road, and seems—as can only a structure that has aged into its background—to be a part of the landscape.

We had driven past the Waldschänke with Herr Zimmermann on our arrival the day before, but whether from its being hidden by trees, or from the dismal sky and the cold air of the day, we had not half appreciated it then. Discovering it now, from the peace and quiet of its sunny rear garden, we were enchanted; we could not resist stopping for a bottle of beer at one of the little tables before its wide-flung door.

We were soon to find that not for us alone was this old tavern a convenient mid-way house for the frequent trips from park to lake and back again. In fact, its *Kaffee mit Kuchen,* either in the little garden at the rear or under the giant beech tree before the front door, were integral parts of daily life for many of the guests of the *Freilichtpark.* Some of them even lived here, having rooms tucked away in the attic with windows peeking out from the thatched roof into the green tops of the surrounding trees.

For not all of the guests of the park, though nudists, proved to be naturists. We later discovered that many of those we had already met disdained to board at the Zimmermann table because they were not vegetarians. They preferred to pay the slightly higher fee of one mark a day (about twenty-four cents) for the advantages of the park and to live and board elsewhere, for instance here in the Waldschänke or in one of the several *pensions* tucked away in the woods of the vicinity, where they could indulge in the hearty fare of meats and sausages popular in Germany.

The primary concern of the dyed-in-the-wool naturists, on the contrary, was the need of living in accord with natural laws, which they construed to mean an outdoor life, exercise, and adherence to a vegetarian diet, while abstaining from artificial stimulants, tobacco, alcohol, and drugs. Because the natural garb of man is his skin, and clothes interfere with the free use of the natural remedies—sun, air and water—they regarded the practice of nudity as an important feature of a healthy life. Vegetarianism, however, they considered even more essential.

The extreme examples were two young women, sisters from Hamburg, who though living in one of the cabins in the *Freilichtpark,* were never seen in the Zimmermann dining-room for reasons quite other than those of the non-naturist nudists. These girls required not only a vegetarian but a *Rohkost,* or raw food, regime. They preferred to prepare their own meals of uncooked fruits and vegetables in their park-hut. Between ourselves, we used to refer to them as the "Turnip Sisters."

And there were still others who, while adhering as a general rule to the vegetarian diet, came to the Waldschänke from time to time for a single meal of the meats that were forbidden at the Zimmermann *Landhaus.* We ourselves used to reserve this practice for the times when we came to feel a special craving for something other than mere vegetables.

After we had finished our beers, we again set out for the lakeside. Crossing the road, we entered a small meadow through a stile bearing the legend:

PRIVATER BADEPLATZ
Unbefugten ist das Betreten der Koppel nicht gestattet. Zimmermann.

PRIVATE BATHING PLACE
Unauthorized entrance into this field is not permitted.
Zimmermann.

Beyond the meadow, within a hundred feet of the public road, was a tight board gate. As soon as we had passed it, we were again on nudist ground.

This *Badeplatz* that belonged to the guests of the *Freilichtpark* was a rectangular field perhaps the length of a city block and half as wide. Bordered on two sides by the lake, it was separated from the highway along one side by a narrow vegetable garden and a row of pines, while protected on the other side from the gaze of the curious by a five-foot and not even supposedly-tight board fence.

How different this from the provision necessary for such a modern Eden on a frequented road in America! Or else, what hundreds of eyes would constantly be glued to the cracks in the fence, and what traffic jams from halted cars along the highway!

The sunny field of luxuriant blue grass and clover was sprinkled over with pink and white daisies, bright yellow buttercups, dandelions, and beneath the trees the tiny blue flower of ground ivy. At the gate stood another *Hütte* accommodating a couple of guests, and down nearer the lake in a clump of trees a double cabin housing four. A little to one side of the rustic pier was a horizontal bar for gymnasts and a small open dressing shed equipped with a bench and a row of hooks for clothes.

Of those guests who had preceded us, two were swimming far out in the lake, a few lounged on the grassy shore, their bodies gleaming wet, and a couple were playing catch with a light rubber ball. We hastened to peel off our clothes, impatient now at missing a moment's time, and no longer fearing to be seen undressed.

How many men are there who have not at one time or another, as occasion arose, waxed eloquent over the joys of boyhood days at the "Ole Swimmin' Hole"? The mud-throwing fight, the dive from the overhanging limb of the old dead oak, the roll on the green grass, and then the nap and rest in the cool shade, all *au naturel!* Ah, what joy and bliss, what thrills! The sensations just thus and so!

But if one would really know anything about these joys of naked days, let him not depend upon dim boyhood memories—necessarily dim when strained through years of memory-dulling work and the stimulations of an artificial life. Rather, let him sneak off to some secluded spot if he live in Puritanical America—or if he inhabit Germany or Finland or one of the Scandinavian countries, let him walk boldly and happily to one of the many nudist beaches—and there, disdaining the raiment of our so-called civilized life, dive again into the cool waters in the costume of his boyhood "Swimmin' Hole."

Of course there never was such a thing as a comfortable bathing suit. Wool scratches, cotton grows heavy and sags as soon as wet, and silk becomes slimy and nasty to the touch; either a suit is so tight that it cuts, or else it is so loose that it flaps and bags as soon as you enter the water. But were the bathing suit not a positive discomfort, it would still come far from contributing to the natural joys of swimming, though doubtless the modern—some say "extreme"—suits are incomparably better than the nineteenth century comic-opera atrocities, especially those that went by the name of "ladies' costumes," complete with sleevelets, bunchy skirts, and pantaloons.

"Under Victoria," according to Leo Markun in *Mrs. Grundy*, "it took twelve yards of serge to make a bathing suit for a decent Englishwoman, and this was in spite of the fact that extremely tight lacing of early Victorian days must have reduced the average circumference of ladies." But oh, the joy of dispensing with even the modern "sun-back" bathing suit! To feel the complete freedom of the naked plunge!

There is a certain sensation to swimming naked that can be characterized only by its quality of exquisite smoothness —the smooth slip of the water along your stomach and ribs, the smooth flow of coolness as though through instead of around your body and limbs, a smoothness that is unbroken by the least hindrance of material, even strap or string. It is an entirely new sensation, one that boyhood itself can not possibly have known, for to the boy as to the happy savage it is too "natural" for him to recognize; to appreciate it, you must first have been subjected to years of using a bathing suit.

And after a plunge and a hard enough swim to make you "blow" and start the blood to coursing through the veins, then to crawl out of the cool water into the warm sun and, with a light breeze gently brushing the whole of your naked skin, feel the water trickle from the hair and run unarrested from the shoulders down the length of the trunk and legs! You cannot resist then a wild dash around the field, flinging water drops as you run, and a roll in the warm sweet-scented clover of the bank. *These* are the real joys of boyhood at the "Ole Swimmin' Hole"!

Soon other guests appeared, come from the *Freilichtpark* to join us. The grey-haired matronly woman and the *Doktorin* got into one of the boats and went far out into the lake. They took turns at rowing and diving, their tanned bodies gleaming in the bright sunlight out there, silhouetted against the green fields and woods of the opposite shore.

Fräulein von Frieling, the pretty little gymnastic teacher from Hamburg, came laughing and shouting, pulling her blue training suit from her browned, boyish figure as she ran through the gate. After half a dozen wide dives into the lake, she immediately started a game of ball, her good-natured bantering and high spirits quickly vitalizing the loungers into taking part. But her recruiting was done too well, for a dozen made the game too slow for her, and her excessive energy drove her to turning cartwheels between her plays. Soon she abandoned us to swim out after three German youths who had begun a game of water ball.

It seemed to be a sort of ritual to keep the body wet. Everyone alternated a few throws of the ball with a plunge from the end of the pier, a few stunts on the horizontal bar with a swim out to the diving tower; naps in the sunny grass were interspersed every half hour or so with at least a wade and a roll in the cool waters of the lake.

A mother and her two children, Gernot of five and his nine-year-old sister—another golden-haired Waldtraut—came to bathe. They were residents of the neighbourhood and came daily at this hour. She and her son had a splendid water fight before she set out with her daughter for a deep-water swim. They were joined by the little Berliner maid from the Zimmermann *Landhaus*, eighteen-year-old Elna, off from her household duties for half an hour. The three formed a self-constituted swimming class, practising in turn all the most difficult strokes.

The row of pines across one side, and the board fence on the other that enclosed the nudist lot, left off at the water's edge. Beyond those points the few posts and couple of wires, extending perhaps twenty feet into the lake, marked off the limits but scarcely screened the view of this private bathing beach. Out in front, from the lake side, there was nothing to indicate boundaries. Adjoining us on the north, no more than a city block away along the curving shore, was a public beach, as visible to us as we to it, where bathing suits were still in vogue.

From time to time boats full of people, some clothed, some in bathing suits, from the big summer hotel two miles across the lake, went by. Often they passed within a few feet of our pier, while we lounged about on the grass or swam within an oar's length of their boat, completely nude. No one seemed to show more than an ordinary curiosity; none was shocked.

Following the noonday meal, we, as most of the other guests, returned to the *Freilichtpark*. Some went there for an after-lunch siesta in the shade, some to spend the time writing letters or reading, and some of the indefatigable ones to continue their games. For, mysteriously enough, full stomachs—even some of the excessively large ones—never seemed to give pause to these thorough-going gymnasts, who arose from the heaviest meal of vegetables possible and went out at once to engage in the most strenuous exercise.

But two hours later found us all at the lake again. There we discovered several people we had not seen before, such as three men, there only for the afternoon, from Scharbeutz and Timmendorf, resorts on the Baltic five miles away, and Herr Petter, a fifty-year-old scholar of Goethe, and retired ship-owner, living in the vicinity, who informed us in excellent English that it was his custom to come for an hour or so every day. *Nacktkultur,* he told us, was of great benefit to his health.

We asked him then whether most of the people in the German movement had joined with the idea of improving or preserving their health, curious to know the common motive uniting these men and women of such varied types and conditions.

"It is the motive, of course, in a great many cases," he replied. "Certainly that is it with most naturists, who practise nudity for the same reasons they practise vegetarianism. Many *Lichtfreunde* have a conscious desire to improve their own health and that of their children. But that is far from being the sole cause for people joining the movement. Human motives are so complex; they are seldom so simple as all that. And of course many people do not know what their real motives are. Frequently they have nothing to do with the reasons their conscious minds assign to their conduct. That is obvious."

"What, in your opinion," we inquired, "are some of the

other motives that lead them into the *Nacktkultur* movement?"

"Well, it may be primarily a love of nature, a characteristic German trait; nature lovers easily come to feel that through nudity they are closer to nature and in better harmony with it. Or it may be a love of sport and outdoor exercise. People may become *Lichtfreunde* because they appreciate the advantages for sport offered by the nudist parks, as well as the freedom of exercise without clothes."

"The enthusiasm for gymnastics in Germany probably has something to do with the success of the movement here?" we suggested.

"Quite true," he agreed. "We have gymnastic systems independent of the nudist movement in which nudity is required for the exercises. Then too, in the proletarian *Freikörperkultur* movement, the fact that the removal of clothes also removes an important class distinction may be a motive. That *Nacktkultur* is an inexpensive form of amusement also has its appeal. The post-war conditions, the poverty resulting from the inflation and our economic depression, account in part for the popularity of a return to nature for recreation. A large number of our young people cannot afford the artificial amusements of the towns, but they have discovered that they can have a good time camping in the woods, hiking through the country, and playing in nudist parks."

"Perhaps if they were more prosperous," we remarked, thinking of American "whoopee," "they would, like the youth of the United States, still be seeking their distraction in automobiles, movies, dancing and drinking."

"More of them would, it is likely. But of course there are more fundamental motives, psychological impulses rather than the result of external circumstances. Many people have discovered that they enjoy being naked, without really knowing why, except that they feel freer, more alive. Man has a deep-seated impulse to be naked, coming from his origin as an unclothed air and light animal, an instinct based probably on a real physical need. Most of us do not recognize this impulse because of our training and traditions. It is suppressed from earliest childhood; if we feel it, we consider it as evil, either as a manifestation of our sinfulness or as a perverted exhibitionism. We all know the delight of children at being undressed—a perfectly natural delight."

Automatically, our eyes turned to where several naked youngsters were romping riotously in the grass, while Herr Petter continued:

"Another motive, largely unconscious, or that we are ashamed to admit if we do realize it, is sex curiosity."

"But don't the *Lichtfreunde* try to keep out people who come only out of curiosity?" we asked in surprise.

"Certainly," was the reply, "if the curiosity is a conspicuously morbid obsession, and if it is based on a desire for an obscene spectacle or the expectation of orgies and easy sexual indulgence. As a matter of fact, even for such people, admittance to *Nacktkultur* centres would probably be the best thing that could happen to them. Unless they were real degenerates, the practice of nudity would very likely cure them of their obsessions and prurient attitude toward sex.

"But the sex curiosity of which I was speaking is a perfectly normal, and in no way perverse, result of our habit of wearing clothes and our attitude in regard to nudity. It is simply a legitimate desire to see what is behind all this mystery we make of the naked body and sex. Most people won't admit it, or may be unaware of it, because of the shame attached to everything connected with sex. This curiosity, of course, is quickly satisfied, and is replaced by a healthier attitude toward sex and nudity. In fact, curiosity disappears so rapidly that, although it is a powerful motive for coming to a nudist centre, it is not a motive for staying in the movement, like the desire for health or the enjoyable sensations of being naked.

"But after all," he concluded, "most people come into the movement through accident rather than any conscious conviction. Friends or relatives tell them about it and urge them to try it. The various reasons I have mentioned make it possible for them to be persuaded, and they are conquered after they have come and seen."

By this time, a couple of mothers from neighbouring farms and villages had appeared with their children, and the youngsters in the park were collecting on the lake shore for their daily gymnastic hour.

For one of the principal joys of Fräulein von Frieling's summer work at Klingberg was the children's gymnastic class she conducted every afternoon, *gratis* for all the children of the park and neighbourhood. And scarcely ever did four o'clock roll around without at least a dozen young devotees, from four to fourteen years old, appearing to welcome her—appearing long before the appointed hour, in fact, to wait impatiently, dawdling in the sand, wading the shallow water of the lake, or turning summersaults on the grass. Their antics stilled for the time the usual shouts of the adults, who invariably gave over their own boisterous games for the joy of watching the brown-skinned little cherubs play.

At the first sound of Fräulein von Frieling's tambourine they came, shouting and on the run, pell-mell, dropping their spades where they had been playing in the sand, stumbling and falling in their mad rush from the shallow water of the lake, and tumbling from their perches on the horizontal bar.

Arranging them in a circle, Fräulein von Frieling gave them a run. Slowly to begin with, then faster and faster, always supposedly in time to the rhythmic beating of her tom-tom, they ran. Then slowly again; now to the right, now to the left; first forward and then backward they hopped around their ring, in deadly earnest, intent on following instructions, growing excited at the slightest trace of failure, bigger sisters scolding and shoving baby brothers back into the line from which they had strayed, and reprimanding them for being out of step.

Next came a series of setting-up drills, with the class drawn up in rows across the field. Here was true individualism; no two of the gymnasts did them alike. Tiny five-year-old Anna, blue-eyed, red-cheeked and brown-haired, showed the greatest originality. It was her forte to do each movement in reverse: left foot forward when her teacher asked for the right; knees straight and stiff, feet uncompromisingly planted, instead of a-tiptoe cautiously and stealthily, like a cat stalking a bird in the brush—Fräulein von Frieling hushing them, "sh—sh," finger across her lips. Anna could bend over at her round little hips, knees straight, and walk on all fours as easily as on her feet; but to save her she could not swing her arms the right way preparatory to an attempted handspring.

Most of the exercises were translated by Fräulein von Frieling into descriptive terms of the movements of animals. Thus in the breathing exercises she had them panting like dogs—which they did most realistically after their run. Then she had them, down on hands and knees, writhingly arch their brown little backs in the manner of a cat; and finally, from a squatting position on all fours, leap like bull frogs, until tow heads collided with bare little rumps and the exercise came to an end with a splendid confusion of laughter and screams from a squirming pile of young bodies and arms and legs.

It was while watching this performance that we, having sidled into the shade of a tree, made an alarming discovery. Our skin, particularly along the arms and across the backs, had a distinct crimson tint. We felt of it and found it warm to the touch. O joys—and sorrows—of the golden summer sun! We were going to pay after all for our day's fun, and pay dearly too if we dared judge from our past experience with sunburned backs. We dreaded to think of the following day.

Well, no more sun for us that day; we resolved to dress immediately. The only thing that gave us pause was the adult gymnastic hour that would soon begin: how were we to evade that? We hated to admit our fears to anyone.

It was Wang who rescued us from our predicament. Approaching quietly he asked, in a low tone of mock secrecy, if we would have some coffee with him at the Waldschänke. Smiling guiltily he said that he did not feel like gymnastics that afternoon, and added with a broad grin that he was too old and fat for such things—which his lithe body, that of a twenty-two-year-old, plainly belied for him.

Gladly we accepted his invitation and turned at once toward the dressing shed to don our clothes. There in two minutes he came to wait for us, himself already in his training suit, which was the only thing he had to put on.

On the way to the Waldschänke we confided to him our fears regarding sunburned backs, pointing out the obvious colour of our necks. But we were disappointed at his hearty laugh. We had hoped that he, at any rate, might sympathize. Yet on second thought, and with a glance at his own smooth brown skin, we fancied that we understood: he, likely never having known the agony of sunburn himself, could not appreciate our misgivings.

Perhaps a dozen Germans were seated in the front yard of the Waldschänke, at little tables covered with red and white checked tablecloths. The men, almost without exception, were fat, smooth faced, and hairless of head, for they were either bald or shaven; and as they smoked their big cigars they talked with guttural complacency across their beers. Their women companions, likewise of generous proportions, big limbed and full breasted, sat quietly by, listening and smiling as if proud of their consorts, occasionally nodding and uttering a "*Ja wohl*" of assent.

We chose comfortable rustic seats at the base of the giant

beech tree, and Wang asked the cheerful *Mädchen* for "*drei Kuchen und eine Portion Kaffee.*" Then excusing himself, he walked across to the brick building at one side of the inn and entered a door that bore a sign "*Friseur.*" Left to ourselves, we sat and listened to the strains of a symphony by a Berlin orchestra coming from the radio inside, to the faint but distinct "tom, tom, tom" of Fräulein von Frieling's gymnastic class that had begun down by the lake, and to the lusty song of a thrush somewhere in the leafy canopy above our heads. The evening air was sweet and still, and across the road the long shadows of the pines deepened the green of the meadow grass.

In a moment Mr. Wang returned, walking slowly across the yard, intently studying some snapshots that had just been finished—photographic work being a side line of the barber's, we learned. As he tossed them down on the table before us, we saw at once that they were pictures from the park and lake, mostly of the guests we had that day come to know, in their *Lichtkleid* costumes of nakedness. To us they had the same interest as picures of old friends and acquaintances.

One was of a young mother whom we had never seen, sitting with her legs curled beneath her in the sand and playing with her daughter of perhaps two. Of it Wang seemed particularly fond, studying it closely and laying it aside only to return to it again. Finally, as though feeling called upon to explain his interest, he said:

"That baby is the same age as my granddaughter."

Out of politeness we chuckled at what we took for an Oriental sense of wit, just as we had at the point he made

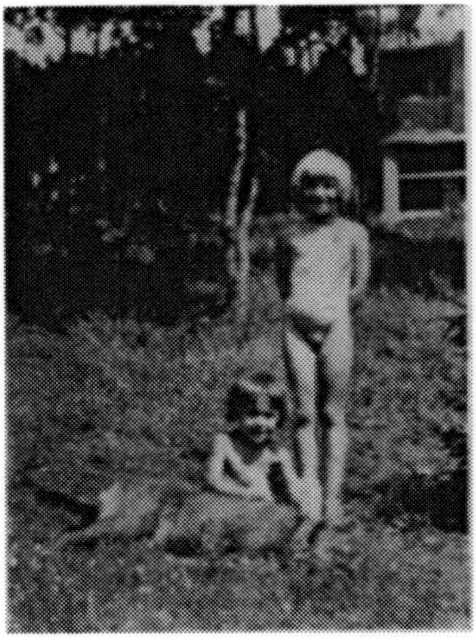
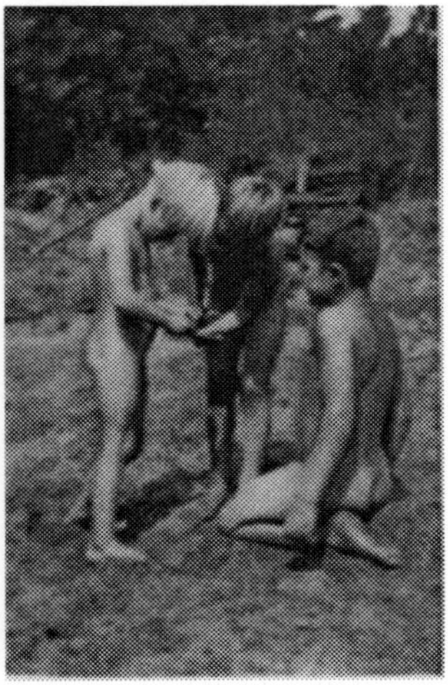
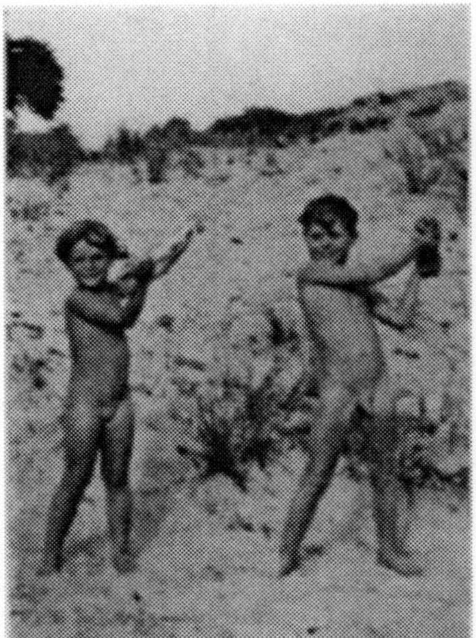
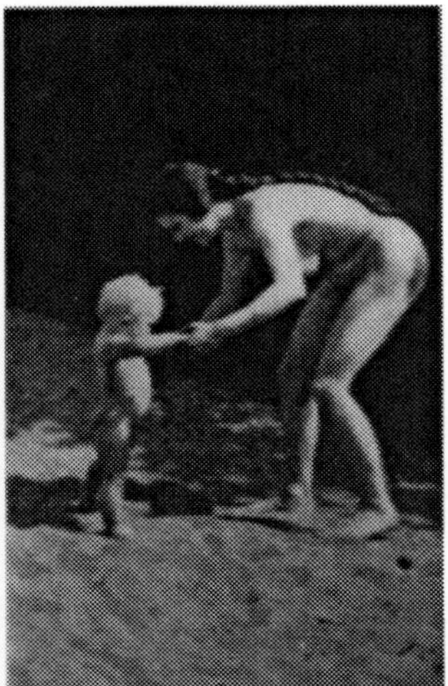

down at the lakeside about his being too fat for gymnastic exercise.

But when he added, "I'm going to see her for the first time when I get back to Shanghai; in fact she's the principal reason for my return," even our politeness failed and, faces sobered, we glanced at him in uncertainty.

That he, this slim-bodied, clean-limbed and agile Oriental, whom we had seen dance with the *Frau Doktorin* and Fräulein Voight the day before, should have a son twenty-five years old and a graduate of an American university, seemed incredible. Rather than a grandfather of forty-eight, he looked like a boy and played like one.

The denizens of this land of naked men were certainly proving surprises in the matter of age. Could it be that *Nacktkultur* was indeed that secret fountain of mythical fame? If so, was it not a joke on Ponce de Leon and all the Voronoffs?

V

TOADSTOOL CASTLE

AFTER THE EVENING MEAL WE WENT SHOPPING WITH Harrass, the huge police dog always lying in wait on the doorstep for someone with whom to walk. We had learned from the *Frau Doktorin* that her anti-sunburn oil, in any perfume, could be bought for less than two marks at "Iduna," a small store about ten minutes' walk up the road. There one could obtain a variety of things, from stationery and toothpaste to oranges and garden seed, including that prime necessity, tobacco.

Although smoking was not permitted in the *Freilichtpark* or the Zimmermann house, the guests might and did smoke on the roads, in the garden, and above all on the front porch of the *Landhaus*. After meals, the porch was converted into a veritable smoking room as the devotees of tobacco assembled for a cigarette or cigar before going to the park. These gatherings were the distress of a pair of swallows which had a hungry family in a nest beneath the wide flat arch of the doorway. They would circle about frantically, not quite venturing to carry the morsels in their bills over the heads of the smokers, or sit on the telephone wires and scold.

When we had made our purchases at Iduna, we were loath to go back immediately; the long summer evening was too fair to sacrifice. The affable proprietor of the store, who spoke some English, kindly pointed out another, more roundabout, way home, a way that would lead us through the beech wood that runs from the Pönitzer See toward the Baltic. Three-quarters of an hour through the forest, he said, would bring us to the beach at Scharbeutz, a splendid place for bathing except that suits were required. After our day of unwonted exercise, we did not feel capable of going so far as the sea, but we took the roundabout road home through the forest, to the great delight of Harrass, who had expected nothing more entertaining than a walk back the way we had come.

Our road led uphill, through land newly forested with young evergreens in regular rows, and thickets of underbrush. The latter Harrass found especially exciting. He dashed in and out of them with a tense air that indicated there was something about the place of unusual interest to a dog. As we came to a small clearing we discovered what it was.

From the thicket a doe bounded, hesitated a moment, and in a flash crossed the clearing. Behind came Harrass, legs working desperately but, in contrast to the easy course of the deer, looking like a slow-motion moving picture. Pursued and pursuer vanished in the brush, but it was not long until we were joined again by Harrass, panting and chastened. He was content for a few minutes to follow behind us.

At the top of the hill, we entered the beech woods. Smooth grey and mossy green trunks terminated incredibly high above us in a feathery tender green, through which fell a soft witching light, such as might illuminate an ocean cavern. Branching off the main road were numerous other roads, or rather trails, buried deep in rich brown leaves that looked as if no human foot had ever trod them; only the opening through the trees indicated the course of the paths. We chose one that led as straight as a cathedral nave through the beech pillars that lined it.

In the evening stillness, disturbed only by the rustling of the dead leaves underfoot, the sense of unreality became almost overpowering. We thought of all the enchanted forests of old tales. This was a wood for Merlin and Vivian, for Siegfried and Wotan—for sorcerors, heroes and gods. German Romanticism was suddenly real and near.

At the brow of the hill we came to a rustic bench facing west in a circle of stately trees. It must have been placed there for watching the sun set on the lake that now gleamed faintly through the tree tops below us. But there were no watchers, except perhaps the invisible forest spirits that ought to haunt such a spot. We sat down, and as the red conflagration of the dropping sun flared through the wall of woods before us, we fell to talking of our day, which had been scarcely less strange than a bewitched forest, and our conversation soon veered to plans for the future.

"How do you feel about it now?" asked Mason. "Shall we stay on a week or so, as we told Koenig we would? Or shall we go back to Hamburg just as soon as we decently can, get our stuff, and go on our way rejoicing?"

Frances was silent for a moment, her eyes fixed on the red sunlit waters that burned in the distance; she was apparently revolving the question in her own mind when Mason, with a grin, added, "How does the back feel by now?"

"Oh, it doesn't hurt, really," she answered, "but it does feel warm wherever my clothes touch it. How's yours?"

"Why, mine doesn't hurt either," Mason admitted, "but I hate to think what it's going to be like in the morning."

There was silence for a few minutes, while each felt gingerly of his shoulders, and Mason unbuttoned his shirt to look at his chest. Finally he broke the silence to pursue his original question:

"Well, what do you say?"

"Oh, let's stay," Frances replied now without hesitation. "This country is too beautiful to leave, and surely the rest won't hurt us, even if we don't dare take our clothes off again for fear of sunburn."

"We'll get toughened to that eventually—after we've blistered and peeled a few times," he reassured her. "If this oil is half as miraculous as they say, and if we crawl into the shade when we begin to feel tender, we'll probably survive. That is, if we live through the vegetarian diet; that's *my* real worry."

"It won't hurt us," she laughed, "to cut out meat for a while. I don't mind this food nearly so much as I thought I would. Perhaps we'll get as used to it as to sunburn."

Mason was far from being convinced that he would ever get used to the food, but he found comfort in the knowledge that whenever the hankering for meat became too strong he could always go to the Waldschänke or run up to Lübeck for a day or so.

"Anyway," Frances resumed, "after a week here we'd be in much better shape for travelling, even minus a few patches of skin. What do you think?"

"I'm all for ultra-violets," he rejoined, "though I do like lamb chops."

Both agreed that we ought to stay long enough to give the new cult a fair chance, and that in a week we should be able to discover whether there were any serpents in the paradise.

That settled, we discussed the question of moving to a cabin in the woods, now that it was warm and we intended to stay long enough to make a move worth while. The most desirable cabin to our mind, the "*Fliegenpilz,*" was vacant at the moment. We promptly decided to tell Herr Zimmermann at once that we would take it.

Without waiting for the western scarlet and gold to fade, we called to Harrass, who undiscouraged by his disappointment over the deer, had been making new sallies into the woods. We hurried toward the *Landhaus,* lest in our absence a new guest should turn up and claim the *Fliegenpilz.*

None had, however, and Herr Zimmermann could see no objection to our going there that very evening, since we had nothing to move but a couple of suitcases. Hastily assembling our few belongings, we set out for the park with the little maid to help us.

Sigrun was there before us. A candle was shining in the *Fliegenpilz* which, closely surrounded by evergreens, was already dark although the light had not yet left the sky.

The bed was made, towels and fresh water were ready on the washstand, and in a vase on the table, soft blue and white pyramids of larkspur. On a shelf over the bed was another bouquet, a bowl of pink wild roses.

Throughout our stay, there were fresh flowers in the cottage every day, brought by Sigrun. One of the first German sentences Mason learned (taught him by Sigrun) was "*Wo haben Sie die Rosen gefunden?*" ("Where did you find the roses?"), which he used as a greeting every time he met her. And it was generally more or less appropriate, for if Sigrun did not always have roses, she was sure to be carrying some kind of blossoms.

We took possession of our "*Schloss Fliegenpilz,*" as we came to call it. *Fliegenpilz,* meaning toadstool, was a ludicrous name for a castle, and the amused Germans hastened to dub us the *Baron und Baronin von Fliegenpilz.*

Our *Schloss* may have been lowly and cramped—there was just space in it for the bed, a washstand, a tiny closet, a small table and a chair—but for peace and privacy it could compare favourably with any robber baron's craggy stronghold. Buried in the woods on the slope of the hill, it was out of sight and hearing of habitations, and far from all thoroughfares.

For airiness too, the *Fliegenpilz* was excellent. It was built of log slabs still bearing their bark, placed upright and separated by cracks often an inch or more wide. The two little casement windows were necessary chiefly for light.

Before we had tried the *Fliegenpilz,* we felt some misgivings lest these crevices should prove too hospitable to rain and insects. But there were wide eaves, a good wooden floor well above the ground, while around the bed, extending nearly to the roof, was an inner wall of tight boards painted a cheerful Teutonic blue. Sheltered from the wind as it was by the trees and the hillside, it remained dry within during the hardest storms we had. Fortunately mosquitoes were all but unknown in the *Freilichtpark.*

As we undressed on our first night we blew out the candle, in case there should be mosquitoes interested in its glow. But a minute later we were groping for a match to light it again; sunburn was a more immediate bugbear than insect bites. In the feeble glimmer, we turned and twisted, examining ourselves and inspecting one another.

"Your back's all right. No redness at all," Mason assured Frances. "But the backs of your arms—they look suspicious to me. Do they hurt?"

He rubbed one tentatively.

"They do!" was the rather sharp reply. "Don't you dare rub any harder! But look at my chest. It feels hotter than my arms."

"Hm-m, it *is* reddish. Better put some cold cream on it. How about my back?"

"Oh, Mick!" she exclaimed, "your shoulders look like boiled lobsters."

He craned his neck and contorted in an effort to see, while she held the candle up before the mirror. It was difficult to make certain of the hue in the flickering candlelight, but by patting his shoulders cautiously he detected signs of soreness and an abnormal radiation of heat.

Conscientiously we anointed all the doubtful spots with cold cream, gently but lavishly, in our prudence even carrying the unction to surfaces that showed no signs of burn. We crawled into bed carefully, fearing the contact of the covers. But our skins so far did not seem too sensitive. At any rate we forgot them in the unaccustomed sensation of a night in the woods.

To New Yorkers, used to sleeping in the glare of electric signs, street lamps, or the lights of the apartment across the court, to the roar of motors, the screaming of horns, and the rumble of the Elevated; used to breathing in their bedrooms the gaseous, sooty fumes of the city; and used to rousing to the clatter of milk wagons and ash cans, or the pandemonium of steam shovels and riveting—to anyone accustomed to modern city life, what balm the flawless nights in the *Fliegenpilz!*

To go to bed under a sky in which the stars burned perceptibly, uneclipsed by electric competition, or with the soft lustre of the moon illuminating the interstices of the logs! To lie in bed and hear on stormy nights the hiss and roar of the wind in the pines like the surf breaking on the distant Baltic, or on still nights, through the gentle soughing of the breeze, the mournful bass of a frog in the *Moorteich* across the hill and the plaintive treble of crickets, until the nightingale poured forth his song, the solo for which the orchestra of the night was a low accompaniment, almost unheard!

The nightingale! Unflaggingly, as long as we were awake, the singer would repeat the clear trills that have bewitched poets from time immemorial until the very name of the bird has become a charm: "nightingale," "*Nachtigall*," "*rossignol*"—a romantic word in any language.

Only once was the song silenced before we went to sleep. As an owl passed over the *Fliegenpilz,* its eerie wail coming so near that we were irrationally chilled, the nightingale's melody broke off in mid-note. Breathlessly we waited through a long hush before the bird resumed its song.

And the mornings in the *Fliegenpilz!* Sometimes we would awaken at dawn, the dawn that came so close on the heels of midnight, to the swelling symphony of birds; we could almost believe that every branch of every tree held a singer. Dropping to sleep again, we would reawaken to find the fissures in the walls golden with light and the perfume of the pines distilled to a sharp essence by the sun.

In a moment we were out in the young morning. Half a dozen steps from our bed was the wood, and not an instant to be wasted in putting on clothes. Postponing our morning shower bath until time to dress for breakfast, we would dash a little cold water on our faces, pick up a carafe, and go to brush our teeth beneath the trees. That prosaic task, a mechanical duty when performed in a bathroom, had its attractions when accomplished to the warbling of birds, with the sun's caress on our bare backs. Not even toothpaste could obliterate the forest scents.

No need to worry about what the neighbours would say if they came by and discovered us brushing our teeth in the front yard, completely naked. Sometimes Mr. Wang did pass with a wheelbarrow of sand for the new path, or Fräulein Behrens, a young teacher who always read in the park for an hour or so before breakfast, strolled through with her book. We called to them unconcernedly, for they were as naked as we. Then we would go to lie in the sun on the hillside above our cabin, or be off for a walk, stopping now and then to greet some other early riser and to chat with Frau Schumann in front of her tent.

Frau Schumann was a teacher from Switzerland who, like most of her compatriots, spoke French and English, as well as German, and who was known to Mr. Wang as the "Perfect Nudist." A tall, robust blonde, she well deserved the title. She had arrived at Klingberg on a bicycle, barefooted, with her tent, and no clothes but the training suit on her back.

A moment's thought of naked feet in conjunction with bicycle pedals will convince anyone of Frau Schumann's hardiness. Indeed, as Mr. Wang said, the soles of her feet were like the bark of a tree.

She pitched her tent in the park, and after the fashion of the Turnip Sisters, prepared her own meals of raw food. Rain or shine, hot or cold, the Perfect Nudist disdained to don her training suit except on the path between the park and the lake. For her, the evening chill and morning damp no more called for wraps than did the heat of high noon.

She told us that during the last eight years she had gone naked in her home, regardless of temperature. On the city streets and in her school, she wore training suit and sandals, but she did not even own a pair of stockings. She was never ill, she assured us; for the eight years she had been a nudist, not a cold, not so much as a sneeze.

But on our first morning in the *Fliegenpilz,* we did not visit the Perfect Nudist. Intoxicated by the forest air, cool and undefiled, and the forest sights and sounds, we dashed off for a run through the park. Around the hill we went, along a wall of golden flowering broom, to the new playground—the middle step of the three terraced playgrounds —and the open stretch of the "Promenade" that gave a view of the lake, a pale blue mirror under the morning sky. Here the sound of the tom-tom beating an imperative summons came to us from behind the trees screening the *Tantzplatz,* the upper playground at the top of the hill. It was seven o'clock; morning gymnastics were about to begin.

Turning, we ran to answer the call to action.

VI

MORNING GYMNASTICS

BY THE TIME WE HAD REACHED THE *TANZPLATZ* MOST of the guests from the *Landhaus* and the park cottages were already assembled, an attendance that surprised us. We had scarcely thought that gymnastics before breakfast would be so popular. The only people in fact who seemed to be missing were the children, whose hour came in the afternoon.

"*Fertig!*" called Fräulein von Frieling, and motioned to us with her baton to step into the line she was forming. Hesitantly we took the last two places at the tail of the line, in order to drop out inconspicuously if the exercises, or the German directions, should prove too much for us—and incidentally to prevent the others from seeing how stiff and clumsy we were.

"*Nein, nein, nein, Frau Merrill, Herr Merrill!*" And Fräulein von Frieling made us quite a speech, from which we gathered only that we were to stand somewhere else.

Running across the field, she took us by the hands and

led us, feeling like unusually stupid children, to the appointed places where, separated from each other by four or five men and women, we lacked even each other's moral support. By gestures she pointed out to us that the class was arranged in order of height, and although towering above several pudgy *Frauen*, a few stocky *Herren*, and Mr. Wang, we could not claim the rear ranks over the heads of all these North Germans, who frequently rivalled in stature their Scandinavian neighbours.

The matter of arrangement settled, Fräulein von Frieling issued an order and rapped again on the tom-tom. As the others advanced the left foot, we imitated them.

"*Laufen!*" the teacher called, beginning a light, rapid tattoo on her drum.

That *laufen* meant to run, we discovered only when we were bumped from behind by our classmates. Scrambling into step, we joined the curving line in a serpentining race back and forth across the field.

"*Schneller, schneller!*"

If we had not known *schnell*, the accelerated beat of the drum would have told us.

"*Zehenspitze!*"

As the tom-tom told us nothing, and our comrades made no apparent change in their movements, we disregarded this order until Fräulein von Frieling called:

"*Zehenspitze, Herr Merrill!*"

Then realizing our difficulty, she attempted to elucidate:

"The foots—the fingers—I don't know how you say; *nicht so!*" coming down flatfootedly on her brown little feet, "*Aber so!*" and rising on her toes, she tripped along lightly, while we imitated her with somewhat less grace and assurance.

"*Langsam, langsam!*" The tattoo slackened to the rhythm of a wedding march.

Slowly, then rapidly again, we weaved in and out.

"*Hüpfen!*"

That sounded enough like "hop" for us to obey immediately.

Then came an explanation of which we understood not a word—something apparently that had to do with a single loud beat on the drum. But before we could call to Mr. Wang for a translation, the light, rapid "running" tap started up again, and we were hopping along at a mad speed.

Boom! The heavy beat, and Frances and young Frau Schoenewald were clinging to each other desperately to preserve their footing, while Mason was rocked by the solid impact of the ponderous belly of Herr Krieger. Mr. Wang (it was some consolation that he too had not understood) had sat down abruptly, face to face with a sprawling nymph.

The line, having right-about-faced suddenly, was running in the opposite direction. The ignorant foreigners extricated themselves from their startled victims to a peal of merriment from the rest, and the relentless tom-tom resumed its regular beat.

At last, panting, we were permitted to stop, and ordered to lie down on our backs in a circle. We were weary enough in truth, but we complied rather gingerly, not relishing the contact of the bare, gritty earth with our equally bare, and oily, perspiring skins. What was going to happen to our incipient sunburns? Nobody else, however, displayed any hesitancy, and we reflected that some of the damage at least could be repaired under the shower.

Our rest period was not "time out." As we relaxed on our backs, we had to breathe to the rhythm of the tom-tom, swelling alternately our chests and abdomens. Nobody whose breathing was shallow or out of the proper rhythm escaped our instructor's vigilance as she walked from one to another.

"*Gut, Herr Merrill!*"

As Mason beamed proudly at her approval, she darted over to Frances.

"*Tiefer*—deeper! Here—*und* here!"

Dropping her tom-tom, she rested both her hands on Frances's chest and pressed with her whole weight. As Frances gasped, ready to choke, her torturer transferred the pressure to the diaphragm, and the victim exhaled, completely indeed, in a wild shriek of distress. Happily Fräulein von Frieling was small and slim. Suppose she had been built like the *Frau Doktorin!*

But Frances's scream was nothing to the strangled groans that issued from Herr Krieger, when the instructor demonstrated on him. "*Ach—Gott—ach—Gott!*" he moaned as she leaned on his puffy diaphragm.

Back on our feet again, we were arranged in several rows, and more complicated exercises began.

In view of our difficulty with simple walking and running, we had wondered how we could follow instructions when anything really intricate should be given us. We discovered to our relief that Fräulein von Frieling herself illustrated each new exercise before requiring the class to perform it. When we failed thereafter, it was not from ignorance of what we ought to do, but from sheer physical incapacity.

Standing with the best posture that we could achieve, feet together—"foots closed" as Fräulein von Frieling expressed it on discovering Mason with his apart—we began arm exercises, easy enough to do in the beginning, but less easy to sustain at the pace dictated by the imperious mistress of the tom-tom.

When the aching of our shoulder-blades had become almost too acute to be borne, and we felt that our arms were on the point of dropping off, relief came. Feet apart, and bending from the waistline, we were ordered to shake our shoulders with arms totally relaxed and swinging loose. As if by a charm, the aches suddenly vanished, and we started on leg exercises completely refreshed.

This form of rest, by relaxation or by the transfer of strain to new muscles, was the only form admitted by our instructor, the sole respite in three-quarters of an hour of physical activity. To be sure it proved to be an effective method of relieving weary muscles. But we were not a little surprised to see this slip of a girl, who looked far more like a debutante than the female "gym teacher" of tradition, transformed into an inexorable taskmaster, demanding as much from the human physique as any husky and mannish "physical ed."

The leg exercises were not so easy as those for the arms, even in the beginning. For while we could raise or bend our arms to any of the required positions, our legs were amenable only to a certain point. Our instructor, however, ignored all physical limitations, assuming, or affecting to assume, that if we did not raise the right foot, knees straight, to the level of our outstretched hands, with arms horizontal, it was simply because we were not trying.

"*Höher, Frau Merrill, höher!*" she insisted, when Frances, with muscles stretched until they pained her, raised one leg sideways at an angle of fifty degrees.

"*So!*" and Fräulein von Frieling easily lifted her own to an angle of ninety degrees.

We were relieved to discover that we were not the only ones out of training, with stiff and recalcitrant limbs. In spite of the national enthusiasm for gymnastics—surely no other country in the world has so many different systems as Germany, so warmly supported and battled for by their respective partisans—others besides ourselves received frequent admonitions and physical maulings. More than once, when exhortations failed to produce the desired result, Fräulein von Frieling resorted to force.

Such was the case when we were instructed to bend backward from the waist until, our bodies gradually forming arcs, we touched the palms of our hands to the ground behind us. This feat, although there were a number who did far better than we, was achieved unassisted only by Anna and Lise, the Turnip Sisters, easily the stars of the class. To each of the others in turn came the implacable von Frieling.

With two members of the class standing behind the victim, their hands clasped at the level of his waist to prevent his caving in at the middle, the fair Torquemada, pushing with all her strength on his thorax, bent him until he had to touch the ground or snap in two. His shrieks of agony fell on deaf ears.

This exercise was the final indignity for Herr Krieger, always reluctant to do anything that involved bending his thick middle. When Fräulein von Frieling laid her brown hands on his pink chest, he wrenched himself from her grasp and fled to a far corner of the playground, where he stood for the remainder of the hour, his arms sheltering as much of his broad girth as was possible, as if fearing an assault upon it at any moment. Whenever Fräulein von Frieling urged him to come back into the fold, he retreated another step, smiling genially, but determinedly shaking his shaven head.

Although not all the exercises involved such drastic measures, there was no possibility of escaping detection when performing a movement improperly. In *Lichtkleid,* with the play of every muscle of the anatomy bared to the instructor's view, one cannot "get away" with the slackness that would pass unobserved under clothing; laziness and cheating are out of the question.

Another difficulty—again rising from the handicap of language—cropped up when we were called upon to perform a series of exercises while lying on our bellies. Whenever we would raise our heads to see the actions that suited the incomprehensible orders, Fräulein von Frieling would call out sternly:

"Kopf gerade, Herr Merrill, Frau Merrill, Kopf gerade!"

If we failed to understand that, she made it clear by coming to push down our heads. As soon as she discovered, however, that we were bending knees when they should be straight, or raising the wrong limbs, she was both patient and ingenious in showing us the proper movement.

Rescued at length from grovelling in the dust, where we had besmirched our fronts to match our grimy rears, we spent the remainder of the period moving back and forth across the field in lines or a circle, with steps evolved from the arm and leg exercises we had been given at the opening of the hour. Only now they were combined and performed while in motion.

First walking slowly, we raised our right legs on the fourth beat of the tom-tom to the height—at least theoretically—of our arms outstretched before us. Then running, we repeated the action, reminding Frances of a musical comedy chorus, only slightly less clad than is customary, and recalling to Mason the less decorative football team, for he declared we were doing nothing more than a drop-kick.

Next came kicks to the side, then backward, with leaps in the air, until, when they were intermingled with steps and turns, we were undeniably dancing. To be sure, only the lithe and supple Lise and the more robust Anna danced well, though some of the others were not ungraceful.

Indoors, hampered by clothing, we might have thought only of our awkwardness and the ludicrous picture the group made. But here we forgot our stiffness, forgot the clumsy, fat figures capering beside us. What did it matter that most of us were absurd caricatures of Bacchantes? Springing high into the sunshine, the cool breeze on our bodies, we were exultant creatures, free in free nature, for a few moments laughing pagan nymphs and fauns.

As our exaltation was dying down, and we were again

aware of tired muscles and shortened breath, Fräulein von Frieling rapped on her tom-tom. A new set of directions: advance the right foot, bend the left knee, keeping the right knee straight. And before we realized what we were doing, the class had all made a courtesy.

"*Dankeschön!*" the teacher smiled, with a charming courtesy of her own. The hour was ended.

As the others trooped off toward the lockers and shower, we ran back to the *Fliegenpilz* for soap and towels.

The outdoor shower bath, at the foot of the hill behind the *Parkhaus,* consisted of an overhead tank into which water was pumped by hand, with under it a shower spray, opened and closed by a faucet. Naturally, the temperature could not be regulated, but the tank was always kept pumped full so that the water lost its chill in the sun.

When we arrived, several of the gymnasts had already finished their baths and were drying off, among them the Schoenewalds, a young couple from Bremen, who were disputing amicably over the family towel. Others, already dry, lingered in the sun and chatted, postponing the time for dressing as long as possible.

Under the shower was Fräulein von Frieling, her dark body glistening in the spray. At the other end of the board which formed the floor of the shower bath, one of the men, a young engineer, was covering himself with lather. Half a dozen others were waiting their turns, and we took our places at the end of the line.

We did not have long to wait. Everyone was ravenously hungry, and ablutions were quick, the next in line applying soap as his predecessor rinsed under the spray. We followed Mr. Wang, and when we started rubbing ourselves vigorously, he asked with polite solicitude about the sunburn, for which we had shown concern the day before.

Sunburn? Astounded, we realized that in spite of all our ungentle contact with the gritty earth, this was the first time we had thought of our burns since the moment Fräulein von Frieling had ordered us to lie down. We examined ourselves in bewilderment. The clear light of day revealed no tell-tale flushes; we were evenly gilded with a faint tan but nothing more. Suspected spots were as smooth as the rest of our skins.

"I believe you are disappointed," chuckled Mr. Wang at our puzzled surprise.

If not disappointed, we did feel a little foolish, like prophets of disaster forced to admit that their calamitous predictions have not come to pass. As we dried, and the three of us took turns pumping up the tank again, we changed the subject by bringing up the old custom of mixed bathing in Japan, where Mr. Wang had lived a number of years while in consular service. But that practice, he told us, has almost vanished now, except in the remote provinces, under the influence of Western civilization.

"Did the custom ever exist in China?" we asked him.

"No," he replied, "but maybe it will some day, when *Nacktkultur* spreads to the Orient."

"Are you going to try to introduce nudism into China? Will you found a nudist colony in Shanghai when you get back?"

He shook his head. "In China it would be very hard, harder perhaps than in America. The Chinese people would

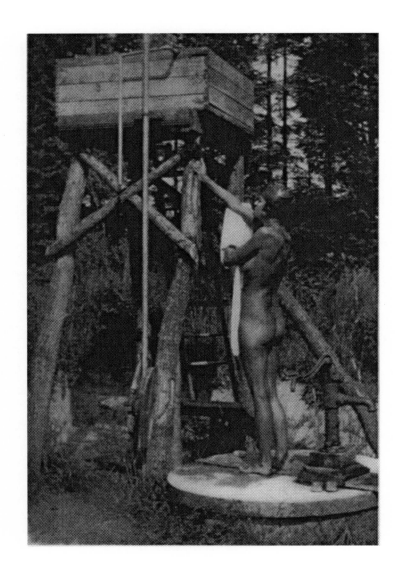

be very shocked, and they are . . ." he searched a moment for a word, "extremely traditional."

We asked him then how he had come to nudism and Klingberg, and he told us that a number of years before, when his health was very bad, a German doctor in Central America had prescribed sunbaths and exercise in the open air without clothing. This treatment had been so efficacious —which we could not well doubt, he being the picture of health and looking about half his age—that when he came to Germany he determined to investigate the movement further by spending a vacation in a nudist colony.

We left him putting on his training suit at the lockers, and dashed back to the *Fliegenpilz* where we slipped into our simple garments—the barest minimum of civilized dress—with all possible speed. By this time, the pangs of hunger were agonizing, and we took a "short-cut" to the *Landhaus* and breakfast, sliding down the hillside and racing through the fields.

The next day, for several days in fact, while our skins remained whole and painless, under them we were stiff and sore from head to foot. When we complained to the merciless young originator of our aches, she smiled:

"*Muskelfieber*. That is good!"

VII

A WEEK-END

AT KLINGBERG EVERYBODY LOOKS FORWARD TO SUNDAY, the day of the largest crowds and the most exciting games, when the residents of the *Landhaus* and park cabins anticipate the coming of various friends from Lübeck, Hamburg or Kiel. Even nudists are generally slaves of the work week and the time clock of modern civilization and can return to nature only during week-ends and short vacations.

On Saturday afternoon the vanguard of the crowd began to arrive. A prosperous young couple from Hamburg drove up in a large expensive car; they had reserved one of the cottages by the lake. Both wore a prodigious number of rings, and Frau Meyer had a handsome diamond brooch pinned to her dainty summer frock. But shortly they were running up the road to the park in training suits, to appear a few minutes later divested of even those and in the one costume that all men can afford. Frau Meyer, who was little more than a child, did not seem to regret that she could not fasten her brooch to her white skin. In fact, she frankly envied the "*schön braun*" skin of the poor typist who was playing *Faustball* (volley ball) beside her.

From Hamburg came also a blonde young mother with a blonde little daughter of five. They made a charming picture as they played together on the lake shore, the mother as slender and graceful as a young girl—a fact more remarkable in Germany than elsewhere perhaps.

A business man from Kiel arrived on a motorcycle. He stayed in a neighbouring *pension* because he could not do without meat and beer with his meals. Groups of Lübeckers walked from the station at Dorf Gleschendorf, some already in training suits, with packs on their backs, others in city dress carrying small valises. There were a few bare-kneed men in the short *Hosen* and suspenders we associate with the Tyrol and Bavaria, and a couple of athletic girls in the brief romper suits worn in gymnasium classes.

There were even a number of people from Bremen. The trip takes more than four hours, but one of the Bremers —an importer who was educated in England and spoke English like a Briton—told us that near Bremen there was no park like the one at Klingberg. Because a member of one German nudist club is admitted to the fields of other clubs, he had joined a league in Hamburg, so as to be able to visit the centres on the route of his frequent business trips through the country. This privilege, he said, was valuable even in winter, for many of the clubs have indoor gymnasiums where members can exercise nude.

The distance record for the week-end, however, did not belong to Bremen. In the middle of the morning, a French publisher, one of the directors of a famous old book house, arrived direct from Paris. Monday he went on to Berlin where he had business. During a visit to Germany several years previously he had been initiated into *Freikörperkultur,* and felt that a visit to the famous park at Klingberg was well worth a considerable detour.

Every bed on the Zimmermann property was occupied on Saturday night, and every other *pension* in Klingberg and the adjacent villages was filled. But the real invasion took place on Sunday morning. People poured in from all sides, on foot, by bicycle, motorcycle and automobile. The *Wagenhaltplatz* in front of the Waldschänke was full of parked cars that overflowed into all the roadside openings. There were even several big buses—or, more properly speaking, trucks in which benches had been installed. The crowd came in families—father, mother and children—in couples, in groups, and singly. There were newly married couples and unmarried young men and girls.

A party of *Wandervögel,* a dozen youths and maidens, were among the pedestrians. The *Wandervögel* and the development of the *Jugendbewegung* (Youth Movement) in Germany since the war have been heard of in America, but perhaps it is not so well known that the Wander Birds often stop for a day in a nudist park on their tramps across the country. In fact, when these healthy young men and women encounter a deserted beach or stream outside the bounds of *Freilichtparks*, they cast off their brief hiking costumes and, without replacing them by bathing suits, swim joyously together.

The Sunday visitors to the Klingberg park represented all classes of society. Among the young people there were well-to-do students and poorly paid workers. Among the older men were lawyers, a judge who had driven from Hamburg with his family, an architect, a couple of engineers, the curator of a museum, business men—many of whom, naturally enough in this region, are in industries connected with shipping—a shoemaker from Lübeck, and an elegant gentleman with a military air who had been Aide-de-Camp to the Crown Prince during the war.

After lunch a Protestant clergyman arrived—not a radical young minister, as one might expect, but a staid elderly gentleman with a goatee. Though it was his first visit to Klingberg—he was spending his vacation in a nearby village—he had met Herr Zimmermann many years before in another nudist camp. He was the fourth pastor to visit his *Freilichtpark,* Herr Zimmermann told us with pride.

We had already had an opportunity to observe that nudism is not incompatible with religious devotion, for early that morning one of the permanent guests, a retired schoolmaster, vanished from the park to walk to church, many kilometres away. The other guests told us that he never missed the services on Sundays or religious festivals.

The political and social philosophies of these people varied as widely as their educations and professions. We found Socialists belonging to the extreme Left, and conservatives who attributed all of Germany's economic ills to the Socialists. The one Communist we found was counterbalanced by a Monarchist.

Free physical culture cannot be accused of being a movement of any one class or party. If there is the enormous association founded by Adolf Koch, socialistic in character and made up of workers, there are also conservative and aristocratic clubs. A fat Jewish banker, over for the afternoon from Timmendorf Strand, the largest resort on Lübeck Bay, insisted that in order to have a good impression of the *Nacktkultur* movement it would be necessary to go to Berlin.

"They have clubs there," he informed us, "that are very exclusive. You meet all the prominent people—the financial world and the high society. It's quite another thing than here, where you meet all sorts of people. My club, for instance—nobody but the best. It's very hard to get in."

He was shocked when we pointed out the *Fliegenpilz* as our dwelling. What Kingberg needed, he explained, was a large first-class hotel that would attract *chic* society people. A corporation should be formed to issue stock, with a board of directors of well-known men. He would be willing to be one of the directors; with his name the enterprise would be assured financially and international capital attracted. In short, he would have us know that he was a kind of Rothschild.

"And then," he added complacently, "you wouldn't have to live in a shack like that."

We looked at each other and at our rustic *Fliegenpilz* in consternation, shuddering at the nightmare vision of Daimler and Mercedes cars, evening gowns and dinner coats, bills, and liveried flunkies with eager palms. Thankfully we returned to the reality of thatched farmhouses, horse carts on dirt roads, training suits, and laughing country *Mädels* to clean our room and bring us garden flowers.

Fortunately, one still meets "all sorts of people" at Klingberg, and there is only one quality that the Sunday guests can be said to have in common: they are all well behaved and decent. Throughout our stay in Klingberg, there was no rowdy conduct and no impropriety. Whatever the private lives and principles of these people in the outside world, in the Garden of Eden they were innocent as little children.

Not all the people, however, who come and go around Klingberg on Sunday are *Lichtfreunde* bound for the park. On summer Sundays apparently all Germans who are not physically disabled go into the country. All day they pass the *Landhaus* Zimmermann: troops of boys and girls, walking and singing; yellow horse carts loaded with flaxen-haired children and field flowers, *Vati* smoking a big cigar and *Mutti* almost bursting out of her Sunday best; couples on horseback; and prosperous burghers in automobiles, those modern dragons still so unknown in this region on week days that horses shy at them.

But the *Freilichtpark* is the greatest attraction of Klingberg. Often at the height of the season several hundred people are there on Sunday. It is fortunate that the park is so large. All the playgrounds, as well as the bathing place on the lake, are filled; but scattered through the woods one can always find deserted clearings wherein to bask and rest undisturbed by the crowd. Even in bad weather there are throngs on Sundays; rather than miss a day, people come on the chance that the variable Baltic weather will change for the better.

Our first Sunday morning, however, was warm and bright, though a dropping barometer did not augur well for the future. Cheerful guests, untroubled by this gloomy prophecy, trooped into the *Landhaus*, the old friends to greet the Zimmermann family and pay their fees (one mark for the day), and newcomers to fill out the application blanks and receive authorization to use the park.

The locker rooms were insufficient. Fortunate were those who could find a hook for the garments of a whole family. Those who had come in one-piece costumes were the luckiest, for they could carry their clothes with them wherever they went. The rules of the park forbade hanging clothing on trees or bushes where it would be conspicuous, but a one-piece suit can be disposed of without disfiguring the landscape. Those who had come from the cities that morning arrived perforce in something resembling conventional street dress, but only new converts had to remove many layers of complicated underwear.

One such couple, an elderly pair, attracted our attention. While his buxom wife pulled off layer after layer of starched white petticoat, *Mein Herr*—grey moustaches turned up in the style of the former Kaiser—took off cutaway, tie, stiff collar, trousers and shirt with a starched front and tails falling below his knees, to reveal the paradoxical spectacle of a nudist in long underwear.

When clothes were removed it was easy to distinguish the permanent guests from the week-enders. Even those who had been coming every week were a paler tan than the dark-skinned dwellers of Klingberg, some of whom were scarcely behind Mr. Wang in pigmentation. Although we were the newest arrivals among the regular boarders, we had already acquired a creditable tan. Our *Lichtkleid,* while far from rivalling Fräulein von Frieling's, contrasted favourably with the pallid tint of the Sunday guests. But by noon even the whitest of the newcomers were at least spotted with pink or tan, for the morning sun was hot.

It was so hot, in fact, that some of the tenderer skinned were driven to the shade. Few had enthusiasm for anything more strenuous than sun- or airbathing. There being no formal gymnastics on Sunday, the only athletics are games organized by individual enterprise, but on this day they were far from popular.

Only the children were undaunted by the heat. They tore through the woods and jumped up and down in the sand pit, raising clouds of dust to the distress of those of their elders who had chosen the vicinity for quiet rest. The youngsters were indeed in their natural element, and we could not but envy them their happy upbringing—no Sunday clothes to be kept unspotted, light and air playing freely on their little bodies, and no obsession with the mysteries of sex. Theirs should be a stronger, more joyous generation than ours. What torments of morbid worry, suppressed curiosity, and longing their adolescence will be spared!

By the middle of the morning the exodus to the lake began, and by twelve o'clock practically the whole population of the park was in the water or on the green meadow at its edge. Refreshed by the cool waters, the athletes resumed their sports with new zest. Whenever a player became overheated, he had only to take time out for a quick dip in the lake.

The Hamburger judge distinguished himself particularly in the ball games by his tireless enthusiasm, though his tall, thin figure, with the stoop of one accustomed to bending over books or papers, was scarcely that of an athlete. The game in which the players in a circle attempt to keep the one in the centre from touching the ball was unusually hilarious; the efforts to keep the heavy medicine ball out of the opponent's hands and at the same time prevent it from rolling into the lake resulted in wild, uproarious scrambles.

Far out in the lake was a boatload of the champion swimmers who scorned the shallow waters near the shore. These experts were led by Waldtraut and Sigrun, Herr Zimmermann's younger daughters, who were as much at home in the water as on land. They circled and cut through the water with the ease of the striped fish we often watched from the pier when they came in to feed at sunset. Just as fish jump for gnats, the young Zimmermanns leaped for the water-ball which they tossed back and forth.

Fifteen-year-old Sigrun was indefatigable. Splashing a ton of water on the oarsman, the French publisher, she darted off like a shark. He plunged in after her, but she was yards ahead of him. Making a wide arc, she swam back to the boat and perched on the prow, a lithe mermaid with her long golden braids falling over her bare young breast and slender thighs.

Three or four other boats were scattered about on the lake, full of old-fashioned people wearing clothes, and near enough to observe that the navigators in our boat wore none. But for all the attention they paid us, they might have been blind.

"In France," said the publisher, "one would make a fortune here renting boats and field glasses."

We had to admit that the same would be true in America,

until the moment when the county sheriff should descend with a warrant that would put an end to such indecent carrying-on.

As we came from the bathing place at lunch time, we found the Waldschänke crowded. All the tables were set, indoors and under the trees, and countless people were sitting and standing about, or strolling past on the road. But nobody was lurking around the cracks in the fence or in the anything but impenetrable thicket that surrounded the nudist beach, although the merriment of the naked bathers inside was clearly audible.

It is natural, no doubt, that the native country people should be blasé, but we were somewhat surprised that this Sunday crowd from everywhere, many from districts without *Luftbadegelände,* should be so indifferent. We saw tourists, anxious to swim, inquire at the Waldschänke about the bathing place across the way and, on learning that it was a private beach for nudists, calmly set off for the public bath house down the road, the necessary swimming suits under their arms, without a curious glance behind them.

After lunch came siestas in the sun or shade, according to the fervour of sun worship. Lying on blankets in the grass, we chatted with some of our ex-enemies about the war, the one subject strangely enough on which everybody could be sure to agree. The men in the group had all been at the front in France, Poland, or China, and the fact that Mason had been in France, although on the opposite side, was a bond between them—all victims together of evil and stupidity.

The air was oppressive, and just as we were beginning to

recover from our noonday torpor, there were distant rumblings of thunder. As the thick clouds appearing on the horizon rapidly enveloped the sky, the less hardy and bold fled to the shelter of the park-house and locker rooms. But the tough and daring, whom we joined, discarded sandals, the women donning bathing caps, and eagerly awaited the natural shower bath. It came in swift large drops, a benison to heated bodies.

In an instant we were drenched, wrapped in coolness and wet, and new layers of water flowing over us coursed deliciously down our bare backs and limbs. Back and forth across the clearings we ran, laughing and shrieking with joy at the stinging lash of the drops. We lifted our arms with outstretched hands to catch the refreshing streams and let them trickle unbroken the whole length of us—down the arms to the shoulders, along the ribs to the thighs, and on to the ankles. The beat of the rain on our skins was at once a caress and a stimulus, and the wet, cool earth beneath our naked feet a voluptuous delight.

With calls of "*schön*" and "*herrlich*" the refugees were encouraged to join us, and when they came their cries of pleasure mingled with our shouts of triumph.

It is clothing that makes rain unpleasant. Even with garments we are not afraid of spoiling, there is the contact of soaked, clammy cloth or leather—a disagreeable sensation and a possible danger to the health. How much more hygienic and practical if one could carry, instead of umbrellas, raincoats, and rubbers, a light waterproof bag into which to bundle our clothes at the approach of a shower. Pedestrians, instead of huddling in doorways like frightened sheep, would step into a sheltered recess an instant to undress, then unperturbed resume their course.

A grotesque picture? Today, yes. But custom and fashion are powerful and unfathomable. We find nothing grotesque, or even shocking, in the bare thighs and backs on our modern beaches, but what would have been the opinion of our grandmothers, who bathed in flowing skirts, ankle-length bloomers, high necks and long sleeves, if they could have seen a picture of the future?

The storm passed, almost too quickly. Revived, as plants after a drought is broken, we ran to the playground and threw the medicine ball while drying off, laughing with glee when an energetic *Fräulein* slipped and fell in a muddy puddle. What would have been rudeness if she had been wearing her pretty silk frock was harmless fun when the damage could so easily be repaired at the pump. Warm and dry again, we had time for more games and bathing before the sinking sun and our hollow stomachs announced the supper hour.

The crowd began to disperse, some starting homewards before eating, others going to neighbouring *pensions*. A number remained for supper in the *Landhaus* before taking leave. But almost all of them added to their "*Auf Wiedersehen!*" a "*Bis Sonntag!*" for the next Sunday would find them again in Klingberg.

And their "*Bis Sonntag!*" we echoed. Our week in Klingberg was practically up, but before the day was over, we had decided to prolong our stay for at least another week. We could think of nothing in the outside world sufficiently pressing to justify our leaving this paradise.

VIII

A DANCE AT THE INN

After supper it was more or less of a habit to stroll to the lake and watch the late sunset of the North. At ten-thirty the sky was still light, even on moonless nights, for the summer sun at Klingberg has long hours, setting well after nine o'clock and rising again before four. Some evenings the bathing place was deserted, but more often than not a few swimmers would appear before the twilight had turned into darkness. Frequently we found the young amphibians, Waldtraut and Sigrun, or some of the guests, bathing in the dusk.

One evening, however, there was only a solitary swimmer, the head gardener, who apparently appreciated the advantages of his job in a nudist park. He swam far out into the golden path on the water, but he was on the shore and dressed long before the orange balloon had dropped behind the trees across the lake.

As we returned, the lights of the Waldschänke and strains of a phonograph playing dance music beckoned.

"Let's have a glass of beer and see what's going on," Mason proposed.

We paused in the huge doorway—a wide barn-door, for the room was formerly the stable of the old farmhouse. It was an attractive scene: beamed ceiling, walls of cream-coloured wood trimmed in blue, with humorous black silhouettes of country life and mottoes in dialect, a porcelain stove in the corner, and in the centre a dozen couples turning decorously, erectly, in the German fashion, but happily. The rosy-cheeked *Mädels* were laughing and chatting, and their partners beamed broadly. All the tables with their gay checked covers were taken by the young folks of the vicinity—vacationists and country people—and some not so young, such as a white-whiskered old fellow who hopped and whirled in the style of the old German waltz.

We understood why the bathing beach was deserted when among the dancers we recognized a number of guests from the park, and Waldtraut and Sigrun in flowered summer dresses. Our flaxen-haired water sprite was dancing as staidly as any young lady in the company. The child had suddenly grown up.

But where were we to sit? We were about to resign ourselves to no beer, when we heard our names.

"Please—Mr. Merrill—you will—sit—with us?"

It was Fräulein von Frieling's English, painstaking and breathless, as though the effort of speaking it had exhausted the air in her lungs. She was sitting in one of the booths by the latticed windows with Alfred Sieger, a vital young rebel, blond, well-built and active, who had already interested us in the park. He was an office worker from Hamburg, we had learned, spending his short vacation in Klingberg.

Eagerly we joined them, and there began one of the conversations of which we had so many during our stay—conversations where by means of pidgin English, pidgin German, and pantomime we managed to understand one another surprisingly well.

The English of our companions was a little better than our German, fortunately; they had both studied in the Berlitz School—Herr Sieger for three months—and had some conception of English sentence structure, though limited vocabularies. Our German was all isolated words, nouns in the nominative, verbs in the infinitive, and uninflected adjectives. In a few minutes our pocket dictionary was on the table, passing from hand to hand.

We talked, as people will in small communities, of our neighbours—the other guests in the park and the weekenders. But our gossip was unusual in one respect: it was free of scandal. Not that our companions did not know enough about the people under discussion. As it was Fräulein von Frieling's second summer of teaching gymnastics in the park, she had had ample opportunity to observe them and hear of their affairs; and Sieger, having spent his last year's vacation in Klingberg, was well acquainted with the habitual patrons. Nor was it kindly feeling that spared the other guests. Both of the young people had a streak of malice and a sense of humour; they enjoyed laughing at the ridiculous in their fellow men, and they had strong likes and aversions. There were a few people in the park whom they disliked, and they had no hesitation in telling us so.

"Him I don't like!" said Fräulein von Frieling emphatically, referring to a young man with a haughty, overbearing manner. "He was *Offizier* in the *Krieg*—vat is *Krieg* in English? 'War'? He is *Offizier Typ*. The *Militär*, the *Offizier* in Germany is *unangenehm*."

Her long adjective was too much for us, and we handed her the dictionary, for we could not even retain it long enough to look it up ourselves.

"Un-plea-sant, dis-agree-able," she spelled out while Herr Sieger elucidated more graphically. Drawing himself up to his full height, he assumed a sneer of lofty scorn.

"Do this! Do that! Get out my way!" he commanded harshly, and added, "That is German *Offizier*."

Obviously it was not consideration for the unpopular ex-officer that restrained our companions from attaching disgraceful reports to him. This conversation was only a corroboration of what we had already observed in the *Freilichtpark*, namely, that it was a barren field for scandal.

The most common fault with which these young people reproached the guests to whom they objected was snobbery, a vice extremely repugnant to Herr Sieger. He was particularly annoyed by a stiff *Herr Doktor*.

"He think we are all *Proletarier*. I am *Proletarier*, and I am *stolz* that I am *Proletarier*."

There was an interlude while we learned from the dictionary that *stolz* was "proud."

"But," he continued, "I do not like when he say '*Proletarier*.' When he say it, he—what is *beschimpfen*?—he insult us. For him, *Proletarier*—*pfui!*"

He wrinkled his nose in a dramatic grimace of unspeakable disgust.

"It is not the real *Nacktkultur,* what you see here in the park. You must not—"

He floundered desperately, in search of words that we would understand, but finally made it clear that he did not want us to judge the movement solely by the people in the park. To be sure, we personally had no serious complaint against any of the park guests, although naturally we liked some better than others.

"In the park," he continued, "there are good mens—people, you say? There are many *aufrichtige— Bitte,* the dictionary. 'Sincere'; there are many sincere people. Yes! Herr and Frau Meyer, the Hamburger Meyers; they are rich, but they are good, sincere. There are others too. But also there are snobbish, disagreeable people."

"Where," we asked, "can we find the real *Nacktkultur?*"

"Among the young people, the workers, the *Proletarier,*" was the reply. "They are sincere. In the *Jugendbewegung* is the real *Nacktkultur.*"

The *Jugendbewegung,* the Youth Movement, was frequently mentioned by the guests in the park, as well as by the periodicals devoted to *Freikörperkultur,* and we were anxious to learn more of it.

"What sort of young people actually make up the *Jugendbewegung?*" we asked.

He informed us that the movement, though started by young men and women of the well-to-do classes, following the romantic lure of leading their own lives away from the supervision of their elders, had become a real movement of the people. The *Wandervögel* tramping over Germany belonged largely to the working class.

"What is the connexion," we wanted to know, "between the Youth Movement and the nudist movement?"

We asked it, however, somewhat like this: "*Jugendbewegung—und—Nacktkultur—was ist*—give me the dictionary—*Zusammenhang? Verbindung?*"

Some in the *Jugendbewegung* are friends of *Nacktkultur*, we were told, and some are not. But the *Nacktkultur* among the youth of the working class is true *Nacktkultur.*

"The parks," Herr Sieger explained, "are commercial. If you have money, you get in. If you have no money, no. But the young people, they do not go to the parks. They have no money. They go out in the woods, wherever they can find a remote spot."

"But what happens if someone comes?" we asked. "The *Polizei*, what do they do?"

"In Hamburg sometimes," Fräulein von Frieling told us, "my friends and I, ve go into the country an ve take off our clothes. Ve are very careful nobody see us, but sometimes the *Polizei* come. 'Three mark,' they say, but ve tell them ve haf no money. Then they *schreiben* our names—you know vat is *schreiben?*" She made the gesture of writing. "Dat is all. Sometimes a *Bauer* come."

"A *Bauer?*" We consulted the dictionary. "Oh, yes, a farmer."

"De farmer, he is very *böse*. He talk, talk, talk. He say *wenn* his vife see us! It is good he see us, but it is not good his vife see us," she laughed delightedly.

We attempted to paint them a picture of what might happen in America under similar circumstances, and although the most essential words were generally missing from the dictionary, we succeeded to the extent of making Fräulein von Frieling exclaim in horror, "I don't like!"

"What about Adolf Koch and his school?" was our next question, for we had heard from Mr. Wang, who had visited the head school in Berlin, of the large numbers of young workers enrolled in that association.

"Adolf Koch is very good for the workman," said Herr Sieger. "He is a Socialist, but he is also a *Kaufmann*—what is *Kaufmann?*—a business man? He has made his school a good business; all Berliners are business men."

Evidently Herr Sieger had great scorn for business men.

"But what he does, yes, it is good for the workers. He tells them how to take care of their bodies," and swelling his chest, Sieger beat it with his fist, his eyes alight, proud of his own strength and virility. He had lapsed entirely into German, but his gestures were interpreter enough.

"And he shows them how to keep clean when they have no bathtubs in their houses. He says to the worker, 'The rich man has beautiful clothes, you don't; you have no white collar even. But no matter; if you have a good body and good head,' "—here the young radical struck his own head a solid crack—" 'and keep yourself clean, wash away the sweat so that it does not smell,' "—he dramatized his idea by holding his own nose—" 'then you can walk proudly anywhere and hold up your head.' "

The fervent young fellow, carried away by his subject and the desire to make it clear to us, stood up and demonstrated, with back-thrown head and flashing eye.

"And that is good for the worker, yes; and by it Adolf Koch does him good."

The two young people agreed that it would be worth our while to visit the Koch School in Hamburg, although Adolf Koch himself was in Berlin.

"And Fritz Bauer," interrupted Herr Sieger eagerly. "He is a good man for you to see. He can tell you about *Nacktkultur* among the workers, for he is in charge of a *Gelände* for air bathing near Hamburg that belongs to the Socialists."

"What else is there in Hamburg that we should see?" we demanded. "Isn't there a school of physical education for young girls, the Hagemann school?"

"Yes," replied Fräulein von Frieling, "a school for teachers of *Gymnastik,* but it is not—it has not to do with the *Nacktkultur* movement. It is Menzendieck—you know vat is Menzendieck?"

We had heard of the Menzendieck system when the founder, Dr. Bess Menzendieck, was in New York a few years ago.

"They make exercises *nackt,*" Fräulein von Frieling continued, "to see vat they do, and because it is more free. But it is hard to visit. Herr Zimmermann took there a Frenchman once, a *Schriftsteller,* and Fräulein Hagemann, she is very *böse* at what he wrote in a book. He wrote it is a school for *Tänzerin*—dancers—and it is not; it is *Gymnastik.* She say it is not good for the school, and she want no more *Ausländer* for visitors."

Before we left the Waldschänke, we had learned—despite interruptions when one couple or the other joined the dancing—that in Hamburg there was a city park where children under ten were permitted to play without clothes, and that it would be scarcely worth our while to visit Egestorf, the well-known field for *Nacktkultur* near Hamburg, unless we had more time at our disposal than we were likely to have. In the first place, railway connexions were poor, and secondly, the park differed from that at Klingberg chiefly in that it belonged to a league—under the directorship of Robert Laurer, the editor of *Licht-Land* and *Lachendes Leben*—and was without living accommodations. The people there would be about like those at Klingberg.

Although it was not yet midnight, the Waldschänke's closing time, it was growing late for nudists accustomed to going to bed at sundown, and the air inside was becoming close and thick with smoke. We left the tavern with Fräulein von Frieling and Herr Sieger, and came out into the night air, refreshing but still, and pleasantly warm. In the east, the sky was tinged with a faint flush of silver; the moon was rising.

"Let's go down to the lake and row out to see the moon rise on the water," someone proposed.

"And *baden,*" suggested Fräulein von Frieling. "You like *baden* in the moon—*Mondschein?*"

"*Ja wohl!*" we replied in our heartiest German manner.

We recalled then that we had no towels, but we remembered that when we were watching the sunset we had seen hanging in the dressing shed a couple of towels brought out that afternoon by Sigrun for guests who had forgotten theirs. Hopefully we ran down to the bathing beach. As they were still there, we undressed rapidly and waded out to the boat, tied at night to a post in the water beyond the pier.

Rowing far into the darkness, we waited as the flush

brightened in the east and the huge disk of the moon, almost as red as the setting sun, appeared through the beech trunks on the hilltop, just above the bathing place. Slowly it climbed, the rosy flush on its face fading to a whiter light, the pure moon-silver that dispelled the darkness in its radiance. It tinted the curling ripples on the lake's surface, splashing the sombre water with flecks of light that finally merged in a broad pathway of molten silver. We watched, penetrated by that old eternal magic, until the "moon madness" was upon us; then feeling the need of giving expression to the beauty that moved us, we remembered our swim.

We followed the silver path back toward the shore, and abandoned the boat for the quiet waters. Calmed by the cool water slipping smoothly from our limbs, the soft radiance that whitened our brown bodies when we emerged, and the night hush, with the Waldschänke dance music a mere ghost of music, faint and far, we swam quietly, slowly, scarcely more than floating, as if afraid to trouble the peace by profane splashing.

We heard the dance break up; voices and laughter concentrated outside the tavern for a few moments, and then dispersed and died out. One group of young people began to sing as they took the road along the lakeshore—fine, fresh voices and true, in lilting old melodies. The singers walked slowly and their song carried far into the stillness; it was long before it had faded away in the distance. We have often thought since of that clear, ringing chorus when we have heard groups of young Americans whining and nasalizing cheap popular tunes.

Back on shore, we became aware that summer nights in

the Baltic region are cool. In order to warm ourselves before dressing again, we ran on the grass, now damp with dew. Fräulein von Frieling began a sort of rhythmic dance, and in spite of the chill we stopped to watch her swaying and leaping in the moonlight, a priestess of Diana, perhaps Diana herself. For the lithe figure, boyishly slim, dusky-haired, long of limb and small of breast, was indeed that which artists have ever given to the chaste huntress.

Regretfully we submitted to the necessity of the late hour and the nocturnal coolness, and dressed. We walked homeward, reflecting as we did that surely the moon of the nudists was the moon of the chaste Diana.

IX

DEPARTURE FROM EDEN

WE HAD COME TO KLINGBERG FOR A FEW DAYS—TO SEE it. We had stayed a month, leaving at the last possible minute and curtailing our stop in Hamburg to one day. We had sacrificed not only such an inveterate habit as meat eating, but several weeks of our long-planned tour, for a physical rest and benefit, a mental peace and joy that we had never found before. For a month we had played like children.

It had been a month of swimming and basking in the sun; of trips of exploration to the old Hanseatic city of Lübeck on sunless days, or walks through the Wagnerian beech forest that stretched toward the Baltic and the fine white strands of Scharbeutz and Haffkrug; of nights when the moon shone into the *Fliegenpilz,* and the nightingale trilled tirelessly by the window; of mornings when, awakened by countless birds, we ran out into the pine-scented sunshine with no tedious preliminary of dressing; of sunsets over the lake or slanting through the beeches of the romantic forest, as unreal as a dream or a legend, its twilight hush broken only by the monotonous call of the cuckoo.

We had come to Klingberg weary and pale; we were leaving refreshed, energetic, and brown as Indians.

The departure itself, however, was not such a simple matter. Leave-taking in Germany, *Abschied,* involves a certain amount of formality. At dinner Herr Zimmermann asked us if we had time to remain for a little conversation and music, as a farewell party.

In the small parlour there were gathered the Zimmermann family and a few of the guests who had been there longest. One of them, a professional singer, took his place at the piano and sang operatic airs and old folk-songs to his own accompaniment, his splendid baritone voice, suited to a large auditorium, making the little room ring and vibrate.

Lost in the beauty and power of its rich, flexible tones, we did not remember that we had seen its owner walk about all day in nothing but a towel across his shoulders, to shade a sensitive skin.

Why should we have remembered it? In a month, the sight of naked men had become as commonplace as men in clothes. Certainly nature's costume is as æsthetic and congruous as modern masculine attire. There are men who are anything but handsome undressed, but are they more beautiful in trousers, shirt, coat and necktie? A tremendous belly is an unappealing spectacle whether bare and unconfined or squeezed into a straining vest.

Our farewell party did not last late. We had packing to do, and early retiring and early rising are the habit at Klingberg. But before we separated, there was a distribution of photographs that had been taken in the park during our stay. Mr. Wang had used his fine camera so generously that his pictures alone would have illustrated several numbers of *Lachendes Leben.* There were pictures of games and gymnastic classes, of groups toasting in the sand, of bathing scenes at the lake and in the shower bath, and of individuals wandering through the park or shovelling dirt for the new path.

These pictures, all of people we knew and many of ourselves, were no more extraordinary to us and the others than so many vacation snapshots of people in conventional and fashionable dress. As nude close-ups of ourselves—Mason shaving under the trees in front of the *Fliegenpilz,* or Frances throwing a basketball—passed from hand to hand, we could not help recalling with amusement our shock when Herr Koenig showed us his collection in Hamburg.

What reason for embarrassment, when nobody was shocked or unhealthily curious or moved to ribald merriment? There was laughter, to be sure, but at those things that would be ridiculous in fully clad photographs, such as the terrible face a little boy of five was making in a group of sedate little girls. And there was appreciation for artistic composition and action pictures that were unusual. When the singer, contemplating the naked portrait of young Frau Haertel, uttered a "*schön*" of genuine admiration, Herr Haertel, at his elbow, beamed with delighted satisfaction.

The rules of the park stipulated that photographs could be made only with the consent of all those present, but only once during our stay did anyone refuse to allow his picture to be taken. This camera-shy man was a meticulous old bachelor, in mortal terror lest his likeness in *Lichtkleid* should be published, ruining his reputation in his conventional home community. None of the others in this heterogeneous crowd had any such qualms. Young and old, beautiful and ugly, all were willing to pose whenever a photographer appeared on the horizon. They all wanted pictures of husbands or wives or children, or of their particular friends.

We frequently wondered that Mr. Wang did not lose some of his urbanity and Chinese good nature when besieged by importunate burghers for portraits of their buxom *Frauen* or obstreperous offspring. For the films and photographic work he lavished on them are expensive in Germany—strangely enough, more expensive than in America, though the cost never seems to deter the Germans from taking their cameras wherever they go. Shake a German, and snapshots will flutter from all his pockets. The craze for photos in the *Luftbadegelände* cannot be attributed to exhibitionism; it is simply an ingrained national habit, and whether the subjects are dressed or undressed is purely incidental.

Fräulein von Frieling was reminded that she had not shown us her collection of pictures from the year before, and she flew to get her album. A few pages of lovely corners of old Lübeck, and the rest of the book was taken up with naked humans against the familiar background of Klingberg. Unblushingly she pointed out her own pretty figure and the strong body of Alfred Sieger. She called our attention with pride to pictures of her gymnastic classes, and of herself bending backward in a graceful curve, or leaping high in the air like a young Mænad.

Frau Zimmermann, leaning over our shoulders, was

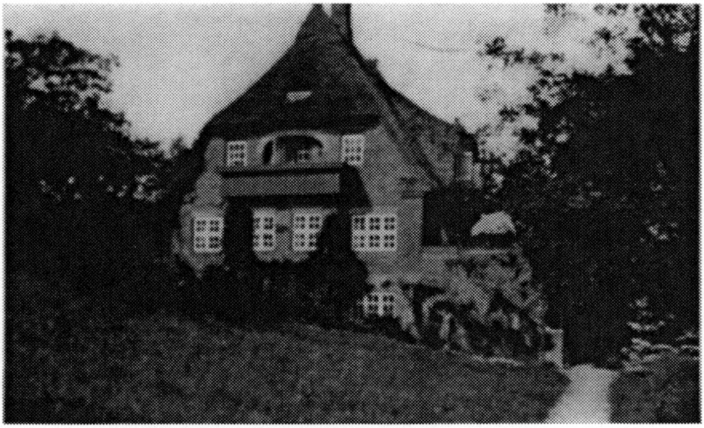

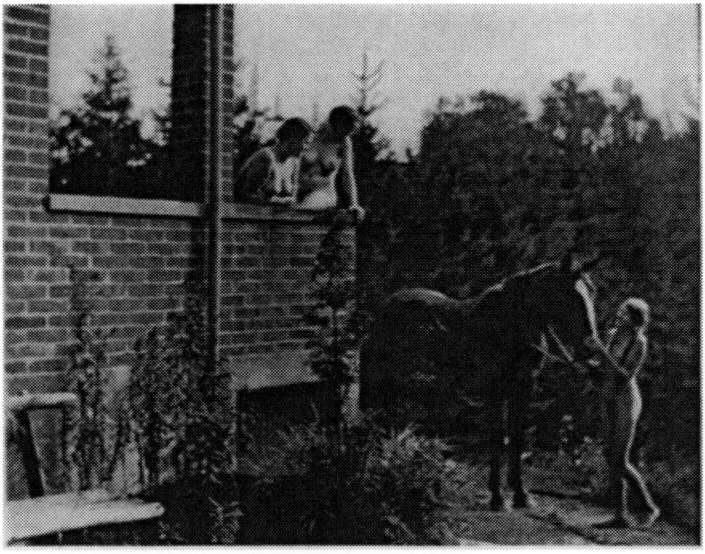

pleased when we recognized her graciously pouring coffee at a picnic in the park on the occasion of her husband's birthday. We thought of the nectar and ambrosia of the gods and goddesses—Fräulein von Frieling passing *Kuchen* made a charming Hebe—for surely beings dine undraped only on Olympus. Some of the immortals were rather over fat, perhaps, but possibly this Repast of the Gods was painted by Rubens.

Laden with photographs—innocent souvenirs of idyllic days, but souvenirs we should scarcely dare to send through the United States mails lest they be branded as obscene—we took leave of those guests we should not see in the morning, for we were leaving before the regular breakfast hour.

The next morning we had breakfast with only Fräulein von Frieling and Mr. Wang, who were riding with us to the station at Dorf Gleschendorf. At the table we found more *Abschied* attentions, for our places were wreathed in garlands of blue and yellow pansies strewn on the yellow-checked tablecloth. The climax came when egg cups were set before us, eggs never being on the regular breakfast menu. And such eggs we had never been served before, not even at Easter in our childhood! They were hand painted, Mason's in a delicate flower design and initialed W. Z. (Waldtraut Zimmermann), and Frances's in an exquisite *Moderne* pattern executed by Sigrun. To break them was positively criminal; but we could hardly set out for Hamburg and France with soft-boiled eggs, even artistic masterpieces, in our pockets.

Then came protracted farewells. Next year we would come back, we promised, if we possibly could.

"Good!" pronounced Herr Zimmermann in French. "And next year you will find more Americans. It is too bad you missed the three who are coming later this summer, but this is only a beginning; you will see."

"No doubt," we agreed. "They'll like Klingberg and recommend it to their friends."

"And one of the American gentlemen," Herr Zimmermann continued, "is particularly interested in the movement. From what he writes, I am sure he will make propaganda for us in America. When you come back, there will be many people with whom you can speak English."

"When we come back," we assured him, "we shall know more German."

Although we did not say so, we trusted that on our next visit, Klingberg would not have become such a tourist centre that the buses of Thomas Cook & Son and the American Express Company would be lined up at the gate of the *Freilichtpark.*

We repeated our farewells to each of the members of the Zimmermann family, to say nothing of two fluffy kittens brought out by Waldtraut and Sigrun—"*Kinder, nicht war?*" Frau Zimmermann whispered to us as she smiled at her two daughters. At length we began to be seriously worried lest we miss our train, so greatly was our progress toward the gate and the waiting horse cart complicated by speeches of which we understood little more than "*Gute Reise!*" and the friendly intentions, and by our own attempts—probably just as incomprehensible—to express our sincere regret at leaving.

At the last minute Frau Zimmermann thrust a couple of

apples into our hands—for our lunch, she said; and just as we were finally about to climb into the cart, Sigrun ran up with sprays of azalea, which she pinned in our buttonholes.

Waving a last farewell to the family assembled at the gate and an interested audience of small children whom we had never seen before but who shouted "*Auf Wiedersehen!*" with no less enthusiasm, we were off down the sandy road, past the Waldschänke, where the barber and a waitress called good-bye to us, and past the blue Pönitzer See. The last landmarks of our Eden dropped out of sight, and we were once more prisoners of civilization.

HAMBURG
NUDITY AMONG THE WORKING CLASSES

X

THE FREILUFTBUND

By the time we got off the train in Hamburg the day was already hot. There were no breezes blowing from the Baltic, no forest shade—an ideal day for sunbathing, but collars scorched and garters chafed the flesh to the raw. We regretted the *Freilichtpark* at Klingberg. Oh, to be able to throw aside one's clothes and stretch out upon the grass, plunge into the lake, or walk through the dark paths of the fragrant forest and feel the cool air enveloping the body and being absorbed through every pore of the skin!

Our friend Koenig being out of the city, it was up to us to transact our own affairs incident to an early departure on the morrow. But they were accomplished in a surprisingly short time: an hour sufficed to change American into German money, buy railroad tickets, take baggage out of storage and check it at the station. We then inquired the way to the office of Herr Fritz Bauer, on Theaterstrasse, to present our note of introduction from Alfred Sieger, the young radical.

Climbing the stairs to the headquarters of the *Arbeiterrat,* or Worker's Council, we prayed that Herr Bauer would prove able to speak English. For we wanted information; we wished to learn more about *Nacktkultur* among the working classes, where Sieger had said we should find it a really serious movement, not merely a form of diversion satisfying curiosity—or even baser instincts—and an easy indulgence for any- and everyone with money enough to spend.

Alas, Herr Bauer neither spoke nor understood English, and his French was only a shade better than our German. However, the fact that we were Americans and interested in a phase of the work he was doing was at once clear to him; he was extremely friendly and anxious to do whatever he could to help.

He informed us that there was a small park only a short way out of Hamburg maintained by a group or club of the Socialist Party, the *Freiluftbund* (Free, in the sense of Open, Air Club), where the members went for open-air baths and exercise on their week-ends and holidays. Did we care to see it—a half hour's ride and a short walk into the country?

To be sure we did. But, it being a Monday, were we apt to find anyone there?

Oh, a few certainly, he assured us—perhaps a dozen or two, though of course we should find many more than that on a week-end, often as many as two or three hundred out of the membership of some four hundred.

Unfortunately there was an important Council meeting to be convened that afternoon; Herr Bauer himself could not accompany us. However, he thought he could find someone else to go—a dentist, for example, also a member and a great friend of the *Freiluftbund,* who would be glad to act as our guide. Would we be kind enough to go meet him?

We preferred not to bother anyone. Could not Herr Bauer merely tell us how to reach the place, and let us find our own way out there? We should be grateful enough for that.

Ah, but that was quite out of the question, he feared. The route being a difficult one to explain, even to anyone who understood German, he could not think of sending us off unconducted.

And strain as we would with our German, we could not muster sufficient arguments to convince him. So back down the stairs and to the street we went, our new-found friend leading us, bareheaded and talking, gesticulating, striving with his German-French to describe *Nacktkultur* and explain everything, his fine blue eyes alight and his thin face—unusually thin for a German's—animated with all the fervour of a deep-seated conviction, almost a religious faith.

We had gone only a couple of blocks on the way to our dentist's when our conductor abruptly halted.

Ah, the *Koch Schule!* We had heard of it? But, we must see it, too—by all means!—in the evening, after we had returned from the *Freiluftbund* park! The Hamburg branch was only a few steps from the corner there; perhaps we would be kind enough to step around there now, meet the director, and arrange for a visit that evening?

We found the Koch School of Hamburg occupying the second floor of an old stone commercial building. To visit it called for a climb up a dark winding stairway, guided only by a fine old curving handrail of wood that had been worn smooth by many years of hands. But, once inside the school, everything was light and spotless—gleaming walls and ceilings of freshly painted white, red-brown linoleum floors, modernistic lighting that actually lighted, not a superfluous what-not or bric-à-brac to clutter up, nothing to impede the mop or broom, everything as clean and neat as in the most up-to-date hospital clinic.

We were presented to Fräulein Elli Adrian, the local director, a pleasant, plain, and efficient young woman in a businesslike office. In halting English she explained the night schedule of classes—two or three sessions five nights out of the week—and she warmly invited us to come see the two which were to meet that evening. Then, after a hurried glance about the place—the gymnasium, dressing room, doctor's examining room, shower baths, and room for artificial ultra-violet rays—we again set out, in the tow of our guide, to see our socialist dentist.

Dr. Schon proved every bit as cordial as either Fritz Bauer or Fräulein Adrian. Obviously it was not every day that an American couple called at Hamburg with an interest in the physical culture activities of the labouring class. But unhappily he too was engaged that day, loaded up with professional appointments, and he discussed the matter long and earnestly with Comrade Fritz Bauer.

Rubbing his thin bald head, Dr. Schon at length apparently had an inspiration. He went into the adjoining office, where we could hear him telephoning, while Bauer explained to us that they were appealing to an architect of the city, likewise a member of the *Freiluftbund,* to act as our escort. But when the latter proved to be out of the city, the two men resolved to call upon a municipal judge.

We began to grow nervous. The first thing we knew our companions, doubtless embarrassed by their repeated failures, would be asking some bank president to close his desk and take us to the nudist park. We had a guilty suspicion that young Sieger had given us too great a character in his German note of introduction, and that Herr Bauer and Dr. Schon were somewhat overdoing themselves in their effort to honour us.

We interrupted with a combination of French, broken German and gestures, to implore them to desist in their endeavours. We begged them to let us go alone, merely to instruct us, give us a map or draw a chart of the route to the park—a plan to which they assented only after a protracted discussion.

At last we were on our way, alone and armed only with a crude chart of the route to be taken and a pencilled note of introduction from Bauer to members of the *Freiluftbund,* our two friends having bid us farewell with an "*Auf Wiedersehen*" that was tinged with scepticism. They suffered no illusions about their own geniuses for map-making, nor about our abilities to comprehend their numerous cautions and instructions.

The train to Hochkamp, twenty-three minutes out from Hamburg, barely came to stops at the half dozen stations along the way; three, five, or eight seconds it would halt, as if grudgingly, and then take up at once its whizzing course, first through sedate residential sections of beautiful backyard gardens, then past quiet suburbs with open country between.

Arrived at the station of Hochkamp, we unfolded our little sketch and fared forth on our journey of exploration. Our instructions were to turn to the left on emerging and to inquire the way to the road to Osdorf. The street this put us on led through a prosperous suburb of beautiful houses and wound leisurely among more and more extensive and expensive grounds and estates.

This, it seemed to us, was scarcely the kind of neighbourhood in which to begin one's search for a nudist playground of socialist workmen. What was worse, the general course of the street did not seem to be at all in the direction of the slow left-hand curve described on our chart. Grave doubts began to assail us.

Nor were these dispelled by our essays in German to the first persons we met along the way. One man, we gathered, was himself a stranger to the community; the next seemed to mistake our questions for a request for a lengthy dissertation on a subject of which we could gain no inkling whatsoever. It was not until we met a small girl on a bicycle that we derived any encouragement; her pointing arm was thoroughly intelligible, and her smile gave us new confidence to push on in the direction we had started. Finally, a road sign appeared actually pointing the way to the town of Osdorf.

By this time we had left the prosperous suburb. There were few houses now, more orchards and open fields of ripening grain or broad acres devoted to truck gardening. The pavement gave way to crushed stone, from which the white dust flew up in little puffs at every step. The midday sun was stifling. We shed coats and hats, mopped our heat-reddened faces, and trudged on. With lips and throats as dry as the dust from the roadway, we thought of the cool waters of the Pönitzer See. Perhaps after all we had been rash to venture forth on such an expedition.

For twenty-five minutes we walked toward Osdorf; it was supposed to take fifteen. But there at last was the big auto road crossing our highway, just as it should according to our chart. Also, a little farther on, we spied the first old Dutch windmill on the right-hand side, exactly as Dr. Schon had indicated with a pencilled cross on our sketch. Our hopes began to soar.

But the minutes dragged. Ten, twelve, then fifteen—already ten minutes past the total time allotted for the walk, and still no woods on the left, with workmen just beyond who would gladly point out to us the faint path branching off to the left—a path such as one must have a care not to miss.

The road now ran deep between two banks, head high, with not a breath of air to relieve the dusty heat. Our new hopes began to ebb, to give way to a new despair, when finally another turn and a dip in the surrounding land carried away the banks on either side; there at last were the woods, though not the "several workmen" to point out the way. All landmarks tallied except that.

Just then the bell in the old stone church across the hill struck one. We realized that the men were doubtless off for their noonday meal. We hated to continue on this road, not only on account of the heat and our fatigue, but because of our certainty that the place to leave it must be near. We debated what to do: wait for the workmen to return—and miss a precious hour of clotheless comfort in the park?—or reconnoitre in the hopes of finding someone to direct us on our way? Desperate now, we chose the latter course and resolved to cross the field to the nearby woods in the hopes of finding our workmen lunching in the shade.

Climbing the fence, however, we found a trail, faint and meandering through high weeds. Hopefully, we followed it; at any rate it was better than the road, for soon it skirted a hawthorn hedge that gave us a little welcome shade. Five minutes more and we approached a group of cottages, where in one of the yards two women stood.

Did they know the whereabouts of the *Freiluftbund* park? Why, naturally! We would find it just around the bend.

Rather than indignantly or in a tone of shame, they spoke with an air of civic pride such as that of any good citizen in referring to his local park. Obviously to them this Eden was no disgraceful thing casting an odium on their community.

Merely a rustic gate of boughs, standing half ajar, and a "Private" sign marked the entrance to the nudist park. No one stood guard; none watched lest the unauthorized enter or the police come to surprise and raid. Beyond the gate, a sandy path wound through the woods of beech and pine.

Not a sound broke the noonday quiet of the forest. Was the place deserted, or was the park far in toward the centre of the woods? But no; fifty feet from the road, along the winding path, we came to a wide flat opening thickly carpeted with grass except on a court for volley ball and on a few spots where apparently games were often played.

Along one side stood a deep, open shed, floorless but with a high cement foundation and otherwise constructed in a substantial and permanent style. A few clothes were hanging on pegs along the inner wall. Evidently, then, there were people somewhere in the park.

Out in the centre of the clearing the sun beat down relentlessly, and there was not a soul in sight. Yet on the far side, beneath a group of beeches, we made out several naked forms reclining on the grass. As we crossed and approached them, two men arose and came forward, eyeing us suspiciously. Without attempting more than a "*Guten Tag*" we handed them our scribbled note of introduction from Fritz Bauer. The signature was an open sesame.

They welcomed us with obvious cordiality. Then turning, they called to others, many from beyond the fringe of trees, whom we had not seen before. Young men and old came out, possibly twenty of them in all, a score of children of various ages, and ten or twelve women—one with a tan-skinned little daughter of a year astride her naked hip. None of them wore a stitch of clothes.

As they walked forth, all bore the mark of great bewilderment. Among them there was much rapid talk, and heads were put together above Fritz Bauer's note. But gradually the expressions changed. We were accepted; all welcomed us, with words or nods or smiles, though still they stared with frank amazement at the strange spectacle of a young couple come all the way from America and interested in their little park.

Well, we must be shown around, of course! But first, we must undress, "*nicht wahr?*" We must be very hot in our clothes—which we certainly were, and we required no second invitation to dispense with them.

So back across the field to the dressing shed we went, escorted by a delegation of fully half our hosts and hostesses. And once there, they displayed exceeding patience in watching us remove, one by one, the altogether too numerous pieces of clothes that made up our street attire. However, we did not mind an audience; we were not only used long since to that, but too happy then to rid ourselves of clothes under any circumstances. Even had their curiosity embarrassed us, we would have been amply compensated in the end by their admiration when finally we bared our backs. For their exclamations of *"Schön braun!"* were genuinely flattering to us, regarding a matter of our greatest pride.

Where and how had we got such coats of tan? (Our descriptions of the Klingberg *Freilichtpark,* perforce done largely in pantomime, must have been classic.) And, what sort of "Light Parks" do we have in America?

Indeed, we would gladly see their shower bath first of all —and, moreover, try it out.

What a shock that cold shower, with water pumped directly from the deep stone well beneath! And what a treat it was to our hot dusty skins! We gasped for breath and yelled with glee as we jumped in and out of that icy spray. Stinging, invigorating, chilling, it was like a quick rest after a long fatigue. And, judged from their broad grins, our hosts, willingly operating the hand pump for our benefits, appreciated it as well.

The park itself, we learned, was small—only about the size

of a city block. But, set as it was amid the surrounding woods, it could all be utilized, not a foot being reserved for a bordering screen. In fact, the limits in some places were marked only by an imaginary line from tree to tree, though elsewhere the boundary was indicated by a strand of wire or a shallow ditch.

Established as a club park in 1925, the ground was rented on a long-time lease; hence the permanent character of the dressing shed, and the cement floor of the shower and the children's wading pool. Besides the large playground, there was a second and smaller clearing where there had been installed some horizontal and parallel bars for gymnastics, as well as a number of swings and a sand pit for the children.

In the woods that bordered the principal playground, however, we were surprised to come upon several small boxlike huts, of far from permanent character, and a number of tents. Most of the latter were but waist high, such as the "pup-tents" that our army men carry on their backs when they are in the field.

But, had not Fritz Bauer said that there were no accommodations for guests in the park, that it had been established merely as a place where the members could come on their Sundays and holidays? What, then, were these huts for, and these tents?

We learned that they were there to house men—and even women, some of them—and constituted in many cases the only shelter for an infinitesimal part of Germany's horde of unemployed. Not till then had we noticed the preponderance of young men among the males of the park.

No, they were not "on vacations"; they were out of work, as also were some of the older ones we had seen about the place. Part of these woodland dwellers had been out of work for months, they said, unable to find jobs of any kind, living only by virtue of the pittance "loaned" them by the government—merely a few dollars a week at the most, a certain per cent of their last rates of pay, depending on their respective ranks of trade. There were present, on that particular afternoon, trained carpenters, cabinet-makers, ship-builders, iron-workers, jewellers, clerks, and stenographers, all lacking work.

Most of these younger ones, since they had no homes and families to support, had been the first to suffer from unemployment. And so they were living here in the park, camping, because they had no money left with which to pay for lodgings in the towns; and from here they were going into the city and the surrounding country—daily, most of them—to look for work, just as all but this handful around us had already gone on this particular day.

Was this perhaps the reason there had been no one playing games when we arrived? Were they too disheartened, dispirited to play?

Of course, to many people the heat of the midday sun was a sufficient deterrent. Yet up in Klingberg even during the hottest hours, there were always some ready for a game. Here, we discovered, there were reasons other than physical comfort for the lack of play: a few, particularly the older men, had indeed been asleep on our arrival; but of the younger ones, most had been either reading or studying.

The Freiluftbund

As we continued our tour of the park, we came to the spots where either this or that one had dropped a book when we arrived. This one had been stretched out here on his belly reading a contemporary German play; the tall, brown-skinned, virile young ship-builder had been seated against yonder tree, before the door of the pup-tent in which he had lived the past three months of enforced idleness, reading a German translation of one of Jack London's tales. Scattered throughout the camp were translations of Upton Sinclair's *Boston* and *Oil* (in German called *Petroleum*), and text-books on arithmetic, economics, law, and English grammar.

At our arrival these young men had immediately abandoned their books and joined the crowd that formed about us. Discovering the attraction now, when they began plying us with questions about America—its economic, social and political conditions—we sat down upon the grass, the centre of a sprawling circle of questioners, to attempt to convey to them a few facts that would satisfy their curiosity. Gradually the women drifted back to their children and gossip beneath the trees, leaving us surrounded by eight or ten husky young workmen.

It would have been an incongruous group under any conditions: they, burning with the ardour of the class-conscious labouring man intent on a new order wherein he would have a better deal; we, painfully aware that our travelling about Europe with no visible means of support might put us in their eyes as among the hated capitalists, or at least in a privileged class with an unfair proportion of the earth's wealth; and all of us attempting to discuss some of the world's greatest problems without even the link of a common language.

None of us having a stitch of clothes, there was not a property of civilization in sight but a couple of dictionaries. For at the first question, we had run to the dressing shed for our small pocket lexicon, and a carpenter had produced a larger English-German dictionary from his tent. But all were too much in earnest to appreciate the comic side of the spectacle, and the lack of clothing contributed, if anything, to the ease of everybody. One barrier, at least, was eliminated: there was no class distinction of dress.

There remained the more serious obstacles: our almost no-German, and their no-English at all, except for the word "solidarity"; our fears of being taken for dilettantes with a superficial, purely impersonal interest in the questions and social philosophies that for them were life itself; and finally our ignorance not only of conditions in Germany but of recent events and developments throughout the world, because during our month in Klingberg we had not so much as seen a single newspaper that we could read. Our companions, on the other hand, were redoubtably well informed.

We had expected to find them labouring under the illusion of American prosperity, the legend of the golden lot of the American worker which most Europeans believe. The unemployed, or those struggling to exist on a too meagre wage, whom we had met abroad had never been slow to bring up the possibility of their improving their lots in America. Would they not be able to find jobs and high wages over here, and would we not encourage them to come?

These young Germans, however, had heard of other things besides the legend of golden America—of our present industrial depression, for instance, of unemployment, and of strikes so bitter that obviously the workers here are not always contented with their lot. In fact their view of America was completely pessimistic. Their America was that of Upton Sinclair, the Sacco-Vanzetti case, of Gastonia, and a supine, chauvinistic American Federation of Labor. And they knew a great deal more about the Communists in the United States than we did; indeed we rather suspected their conception of the magnitude of Soviet activities here resembled that of a former Police Commissioner of New York City.

Most painful of all was our attempt, with only a vague and superficial acquaintance with German Socialism, to explain the difference between the Socialist Party in America and that in Germany. To discuss matters of which one knows little, in a language one knows not at all, is exhausting—almost as exhausting as a tramp from Hamburg to the park of the *Freiluftbund*. Hence we were not altogether sorry when a gathering on the playground indicated that the conversation was to be interrupted by games.

For, as if by some prearrangement, and by way of showing their American guests that they were not averse to play, the others had emerged from their bowery retreats. A slim young woman of possibly twenty-two, with a beautiful bronzed body—a jobless stenographer—organized a game of volley ball. In it she gave places to a grey-haired and stooped old cabinet-maker, and to the mother of the one-year-old child. The latter, deposited to play on a blanket in the sun, was being watched over by a dark-skinned woman whose big stomach and fat thighs were but poorly covered by the red sweater that she was knitting in the nearby shade.

Three men, perhaps too heavy to play such an active game as volley ball but hoping to reduce their ponderous paunches, began tossing a heavy medicine ball, executing first one and then another of all the most difficult passes—with the right hand alone, the left hand, backward over the head, between the legs, etc. And on the opposite side of the clearing a smaller group commenced still another kind of a game.

We ourselves felt no need for exercise. Our hike out there from Hamburg through the heat and dust had quite sufficed, especially since we had arisen at an early hour in Klingberg that morning and had not found time for lunch. We trusted, therefore, that we might be allowed merely to watch the others. But apparently something more was expected of us.

So volley ball it was—and a gruelling half-hour's game, too—for the sake of the American reputation for sport, we told ourselves. Then, pleading the need of an early return to the city, we had a second shower of icy water straight from the pump, and fifteen minutes on the sunny grass to dry off.

How we hated to don again our clothes! But it was nothing compared to putting on our shoes. For, *mein Gott,* the blisters we discovered on our feet! Obviously a month's barefoot bliss had ill prepared our feet for a dusty hike in shoes. It was positive torture for us to walk. But there were no taxicabs waiting at the gate of this workmen's park, nor

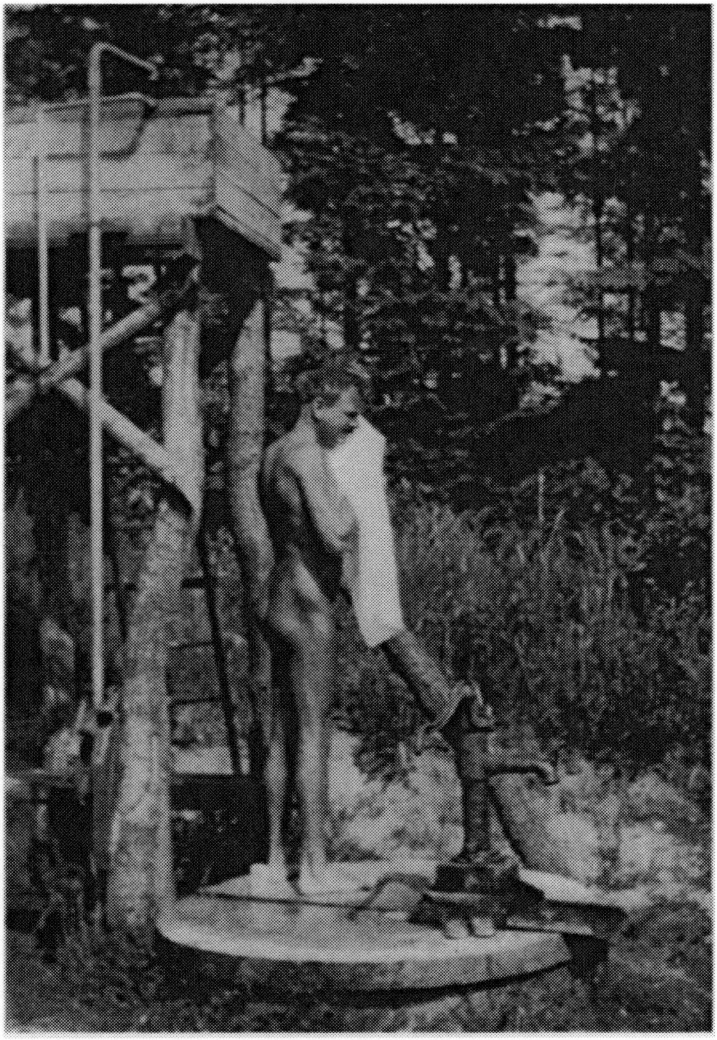

streetcars to take us to the interurban station at Hochkamp; nothing remained for us but to hobble back.

That return trip still lives in our memories as a terrible nightmare. It seemed that our slow pace along that winding road would never bring us to the end. And after we were aboard the train, our feet swelled until we feared they would burst our shoes.

Our agony had quite eclipsed the memory of our evening's plans. It was not till we were back in our hotel and had had a few minutes' rest that we recalled the Koch School and the arrangements already made for our visit there. The mere thought of it then made us despair.

Well, we simply could not go. We would go out in a little bit for a bite to eat, and then come back and pile in bed; that was the only sensible thing for us to do.

And yet, Fräulein Adrian would surely be expecting us; so perhaps would be Fritz Bauer. For he had said that he would meet us there if he found it possible to finish his affairs. Could we fail to put in an appearance there after all the time and attention they had given us? Were we not rather obliged to go?

XI

THE KOCH SCHULE

FOOT BATHS HELPED, AS DID A CHANGE OF SHOES. WE limped out and down the street. A cold glass of beer, a hasty meal, and we turned toward the *Koch Schule,* exactly an hour late of the appointed time. It was a secret joy to think that we had missed one class, and we hoped to be able to cut the other short. Our only real interest was in our hotel and bed.

Fräulein Elli Adrian, busy as a big executive but not so curt, received us with a cordial smile. She informed us that the first class—as we had hoped—was through, and that the second would soon begin. Then introducing us, she turned us over to Herr Heiner Oppermann, the teacher that evening, a happy, animated young man of perhaps twenty-four, who was sockless, in "shorts," sandals, and a waist-length leathern jacket with brass buttons down the front.

Alas, he did not speak English. Nevertheless he made us understand that we might follow him to the dressing room —and our resistance was too low by then, our reactions too tardy, for us to think of explaining that all we wanted was chairs in which to sit quietly by and watch.

The dressing room, small to begin with, was packed with young people, men and women together, either completely naked or in the act of dressing or undressing. At least twenty or thirty were there, most of them in their late teens or early twenties, all of them laughing and talking, the group from the first class of the evening putting on their clothes for departure, the rest taking off theirs preparatory to the session that was to follow. The place rang with the echoes of happiness, good spirits and camaraderie, everybody addressing the others as "Heinz" or "Fritz" or "Anna" or "Hilda," and by the familiar form of "*du*"—a common practice, we were told, in all the Koch schools of Germany.

Along the two sides of the little room ran low wooden benches, upon the wall above each a row of hooks for clothes. With a wave of his hand and a gracious smile Herr Oppermann invited us to a single space on the nearest bench, the only seat available; at the same instant, Fräulein Adrian appeared at the door with two bath towels and a lady's bathing cap.

It was clear that we were expected to bathe. However, we surmised this was one of the rituals of the place, a thing which everyone did as automatically as a Turk sheds his shoes at the door of his mosque. And anyway, we told ourselves, a good hot bath could do no harm; it might even relieve some of our weariness.

Slowly we edged into the crowded room, now squeezing our way around a good-looking young woman of twenty-two or three who was occupied in hooking her brassière, and now behind a naked young man who hopped about on one foot while he dried the other with a towel.

Suddenly a hush fell upon the room. All eyes were turned on us, and we heard "*Amerikaner*" whispered once or twice. Apparently our coming had been foretold. A tall naked youth, seated to pull on his socks, got up and proffered us his place. At our essayed "*Dankeschön*" all laughed, and some in good-humoured irony exclaimed, "*Ach, sie sprechen Deutsch!*" All eyes now were friendly eyes; smiles welcomed us. We took our seats and began to unfasten shoes.

At this moment another girl appeared in the door. Arms raised to pull a towel across her back, her firm round breasts still glistening wet, she paused just inside and smilingly surveyed the scene. The last of the earlier class to come from the shower across the hall, she was the signal for the second group to begin their baths. Two husky youths, already undressed, started forward with a bound. As they rushed through the door, they playfully jostled her, when quick as a flash she turned and snapped her wet towel on their retreating backs, much to the delight of everyone, even the victims themselves, who paused across the hall and turned to grin.

As we proceeded to undress, others, boys and girls together, finished and left for the shower room whence, at every opening of the door, came the hiss of spraying water and mixed voices raised in song. The laughter and high spirits of the place were irresistible; our own pulses beat faster, and temporarily we forgot our fatigue.

For the second time that day the discarding of our clothes elicited sweet flattery. As we disclosed our bronzed backs and limbs, our companions arrested for the moment their own concern with clothes to gather around us and admire the smooth colour of our skins. "*Ach, sehr schön!*" and "*Herrlich!*" some of them exclaimed.

And their remarks had a patent sincerity when we learned that most of these young people, being still in school or else engaged in unremunerative apprenticeships, but rarely got out even to the park of the *Freiluftbund*. While the artificial ultra-violet rays of the lamps in the adjoining room were beneficial and far better than none, they did not tan the skin as do the open air and sun. Hence these youngsters envied us, and expressed their envy candidly.

Again the same questions about where and how we had acquired such brown; and again the inevitable queries regarding such things as "Light Parks" in America.

The shower baths, first hot then cold, did wonders for us; they soothed and seemed to wash away some of the lameness of our bones. The last ones in, we dallied there, reluctant to leave the sweet sting of the spray, until at the door Herr Oppermann appeared, stuck in his smiling countenance, and shouted "*Komme!*" Hastily drying ourselves, we stepped again into the hall just as he came bounding by, beating a tom-tom to call his class. With another flashing smile and "*Komme!*" he went on in the direction of the gymnasium. We followed more leisurely, delighting in the smooth coolness of the waxed linoleum floor upon our blistered feet.

A class of eleven was already there, seven men and four women, all young and nude, wearing not so much as a pair of shoes. Herr Oppermann alone was clad. The room itself, now that we had time to look at it, was small, high-ceilinged, and wholly bare: not a single piece of gymnastic equipment, not a picture or decoration on the walls. Except for the red linoleum floor and two sets of dark heavy drapes at the windows that looked down on the street, everything, including the high porcelain stove in the corner, was spotless white.

At a resounding tattoo on the drum, the class arranged itself in a circle about the room. Again smiling with his manifest amiability, Herr Oppermann motioned us to places in the ring.

What did this mean? participate? We had not brought our weary bodies there for that. We were there merely to look on. But, we thought, this was not the time for us to explain to him, especially by a slow and dubious process of pantomime; better to make a start, at least, and then drop out. We could soon retire to a corner of the room, and surely this young man would understand.

The orders, being in German naturally, meant nothing to us; we had simply to watch and imitate the other members of the class. Taking long strides, on our toes, we began circling the room to the slow beat of the tom-tom. At first slowly, very slowly—like the movement of a slow-motion picture film, Herr Oppermann chanting his instructions to the rhythm of his drum—then faster, and faster still, we went, round and round the little room, madly, running until we were ready to drop in our tracks from sheer exhaustion. Then, just as gradually slowing our pace, we at last stopped and, at a final thump of the tom-tom by Oppermann, threw ourselves panting on the floor. Lying there flat upon our backs, we stretched wide our arms and legs to rest, while our chests and stomachs rose and fell to heaving breaths.

Three minutes were the allotted time for rest. It was surprising how that sufficed for one to regain his breath. Scarcely half of it had passed when everyone was sitting up.

Just then another youth came in, late, and was greeted with a chorus of joyful shouts; apparently this tall Hans was a favourite. Again there was laughter, jokes on every side. Some commenced performing tricks. One youth rolled backward until, standing on the nape of his neck, legs and trunk pointing straight toward the ceiling, he "peddled the bicycle" in the air. Hans, the late-comer, proceeded to walk about the room on his hands, patting his companions from time to time on their heads with his feet. Then one of the girls put all the boys to shame by "doing the splits," first forwards and then sideways.

Nor were any of these things done in the manner of stunts, in the spirit of "showing off." It was simply that these young people were too full of life and healthy energy to rest quietly for three whole minutes; this was merely their way of having fun. In fact, but for an occasional furtive glance, when their curiosity would reassert itself, they seemed utterly oblivious of us.

At the first rap of Herr Oppermann's drum, all were up and in their places again. We followed their example, forced by a pride that was stronger than our inertia of fatigue, determined to stay with them long enough to prove that we were no weaklings, feeling that proof was necessary since we could not explain our weariness.

There followed some back and arm exercises, similar to those of an army setting-up drill: thrusting of arms forward and sidewise, first over the head, then downward along the sides; touching the hands to the floor without bending the knees; and describing circles first with the head, then with the body above the waist.

This was less painful to blistered feet; we even felt that perhaps we could still last a while. So we kept the places assigned to us, following the other members of the class through various movements, in combination and sequence, always to the rhythmic beating drum, the clapping hands, and the singing count of Herr Oppermann, who either stood in a corner stamping time with his foot, or else pranced along the walls of the room offering criticisms and encouragement.

During the rest period that followed, a lively argument arose over one of the exercises we had just been given. Several of the students were frankly critical, offering suggestions to the instructor as freely as though to one of their own number. Also they addressed him, we noticed, as "*du,*" just as they did each other. Although unconvinced by their arguments, Herr Oppermann was willing to try their proposed changes. So at the end of the rest period, we repeated the exercise in the manner suggested, whereupon the young instructor wholeheartedly agreed that it worked out much better, and said that henceforth he would use their method.

Next we were made to lie on our backs, all our feet pointing toward the centre of the ring, where Oppermann stationed himself. In this position we were commanded to wave our legs—first one, then both—up to the vertical and out to the side, slowly and to the count; then to describe circles in the air with the toes. We were next told to cross our arms over our chests and to raise from the floor first our heads, then our shoulders, then feet, and—by rounding the back—"do a rocking horse." And, turning over onto our bellies, clasping the arms behind our backs, we were told to do the same thing on our stomachs—or, at least, try.

Following another rest, the class retired against the walls while two at a time were taken to the centre of the floor to perform an amazing roll. From a sitting position, knees raised and spread so that the heels were close drawn in, we were instructed to reach down between the legs and, clasping the toes between our hands, pull the feet from the floor. Then pushing us over so that we lay upon our sides, Herr Oppermann made us roll across our backs, past the other side, and on up to a sitting position again. Thus, by repeating the sequence, we each described an elliptical path upon the floor—not an impossible feat once the trick was learned.

The rub came when one failed to roll with sufficient force across the back to carry him past his side and on up to the erect again. For, lacking momentum enough for that, he could not rise so long as he held his feet, but wobbled around like an awkward Junebug on its back. Strain as one would the sole effect was to pull the feet higher and spread wider the legs—a most undignified posture, particularly for a lady.

Before we knew it, the hour was up. We were both surprised and proud to find that we had lasted it out. Most amazing of all, however, was the way we felt. We had begun it as though starting some terrible ordeal; we finished it actually feeling refreshed.

The class being dismissed, there was another mad rush for the baths, and though there were no handicaps given for sex, not all the winners were masculine.

The half dozen showers—three each on two sides of the tiny square room, with no partition or pretence of the least privacy—nicely accommodated eight or ten, some using the sprays while others soaped up at one side. In a corner a young man was lathering a girl's back, a favour that she afterwards returned. Again there was joking and laughter, but that soon gave way to song in which all joined with fine lusty harmony.

It seems that the German people must sing, both while they work and while they play. Witness the *Wandervögel*, who sing their way along all the highroads of the countryside. No wonder, then, that song should here drown out the hissing water of the shower room, when even American men—if they never sing elsewhere—lift their voices in their morning baths.

Following our shower we were led down the hall to another small square room. There, lying side by side on a row of low white cots, were our recent classmates—still unadorned except for goggles worn to protect their eyes—their white young bodies whiter yet under the glare of light that flooded them from a battery of ultra-violet lamps above. Some were on their backs, legs outstretched and arms thrown above their heads; some on their sides as if asleep; still others lay on their bellies, to expose their spines to the violet rays. At last they were silent, for the first time since we had met them that evening—silent and relaxed, the exuberance of their healthy youth finally quiescent. A poor substitute, perhaps, this artificial light, for the open air and sun of the out-of-doors, but better by far than no light at all.

We had now spent an hour and a half in this Koch School;

we had seen young men and women meet and mingle and play and bathe and rest together, all devoid of clothes, without so much as a sign of a single improper act, without the least trace of an unhealthy thought, and—most significant of all—without a symptom of any of the manifold inhibitions so commonly the result of adolescent sex consciousness. There was about the place itself, as about everyone we had seen in it, pupils and teachers alike, an air of cleanliness, moral as well as physical, of happy health of body and mind.

It had all proved a great illumination for us, a thing quite beyond our most extravagant hopes, not to say expectations. Nothing comparable to it had ever been seen or even heard of by either of us before. We fell to wondering what would be the result if something of the same sort were attempted in America, say in New York, Chicago, Philadelphia, or Boston—what, that is, besides the immediate arrest of whosoever proposed it, probably before ever the thing had been so much as tried, and his conviction for contributing to the delinquency of youths?

But suppose it were given an actual trial in the United States, what would probably be the reaction, resulting from our Puritanical heritage, of even the pick of our own Young America—the cream, the soundest physically and mentally, of the stenographers, let us say, and the clerks, accountants, mechanics, and what-not? Would they be apt to conduct themselves in the same manner as had these young Germans? Or would they break themselves up with ingrained inhibitions as a consequence of our traditional taboos? And what might be the form coming out of that break-up—a cold lifeless apathy, an asexuality, or would it be anarchy?

Finally dressed again, we sought out Fräulein Adrian in her office, anxious to learn more about the Koch schools. There we found her, at nearly ten o'clock, still diligently at work, for the activities of the Koch schools involve more than gymnastic instruction and the correspondence, records and accounts necessary in any institution. The Koch organization gives lectures and publishes various magazines and books of an educational nature dealing with physical culture, hygiene, and social and ethical questions. But immediately she pushed all aside to welcome us and graciously proceeded to answer every question that we could ask. Moreover, she equipped us with a small library of literature on the work that she and her organization had done and were doing.

She told us, for instance, that hers was but one of the six Koch schools in Germany, that there were others in Barmen-Eberfeld, Breslau, Ludwigshafen, and Mannheim, besides the main and original school in Berlin. Also, in conjunction with the Berlin school, there was a teacher's seminary offering special studies in such subjects as anatomy, psychology, sociology, teaching methods, massage, etc.—a three to four years' course calling for eighteen to twenty hours of study a week.

We learned that a student, on completing this course in the seminary, must have a year or more of experience in actual teaching before he is qualified for a directorship in a *Koch Schule*. Thus Herr Oppermann, for example, having graduated with a diploma from the seminary, was spending a year in Hamburg as Fräulein Adrian's assistant, preparatory to the next year when he himself expected to be the director of a school.

But, according to the information given us by Fräulein Adrian, the most unique feature of the Koch schools is their relationship with the pupils enrolled in them. We had already had occasion to note the habitual use of the familiar "*du*" by both pupils and teachers, an outward sign of the relationship of complete equality at which they aim. But apparently the socialism of the Koch schools goes deeper than any mere outward symbol.

In return for the gymnastic training, the medical attention, the lectures, and the supervised study which comprise the principal work of the Koch schools, the students, or "members," pay no specified matriculation fee, no arbitrary sum of money. Instead, they contribute five per cent of their incomes, whatever that may be. If, therefore, a student has no income, instead of being dropped from the rolls of the school, he continues to receive the full benefits of his membership without himself contributing anything until he begins to earn again.

It was on account of this provision, Fräulein Adrian told us, that the Koch schools in Germany have been having financial difficulties recently. For with the widespread unemployment of the country, so many of the pupils have been out of work, and hence out of incomes, that the revenues of the schools have been greatly diminished without any corresponding decrease in cost of operation.

As to the story of how the Koch schools came to be started, however, we gained scant satisfaction from our interview that evening; in that instance the difficulties of language proved too great. It was not until some time later that we discovered, in one of the pamphlets Fräulein Adrian had given us—*Freie Körperkultur in Wort und Bild*—the reprint of a newspaper account that appeared in *Vorwärts* (Berlin), November 27, 1929.

According to it, the founder of the institution, Adolf Koch, a young professor, decided one day—it was back during the painful period of Germany's monetary inflation—to come to the aid of the undernourished and sickly children of Berlin. With this in view he gathered together a group of young teachers for the purpose of educating the students according to an entirely new principle of nude exercise in the open air and sun. The children took to this method quickly and evinced great joy in doing the exercises. But one day a prudish woman entered the school while Professor Koch was drilling his pupils in their state of paradisical simplicity.

Uttering a cry of heresy, she mobilized the clergy, appealed to the modesty of well-thinking people, and the affair terminated in a sensational suit in the courts. The clerical and bourgeois press published vituperative articles under such headings as "Nude Dances in the School." But the suit ended with a reprimand for Adolf Koch because, according to a statute dating from 1752, permission to use school property for private purposes had to be obtained not only from the school inspector—which had been done—but also from the provincial board of education.

With this began the campaign for proletarian *Nacktkultur*. And according to the *Vorwärts* account, the Koch gymnastic method is today as officially recognized by the German state as any other system. This fact is perhaps attested by the character of the three-day "Congress" on

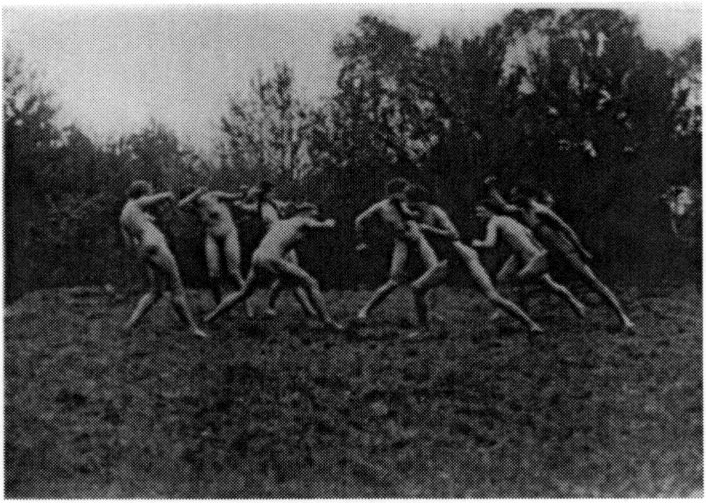

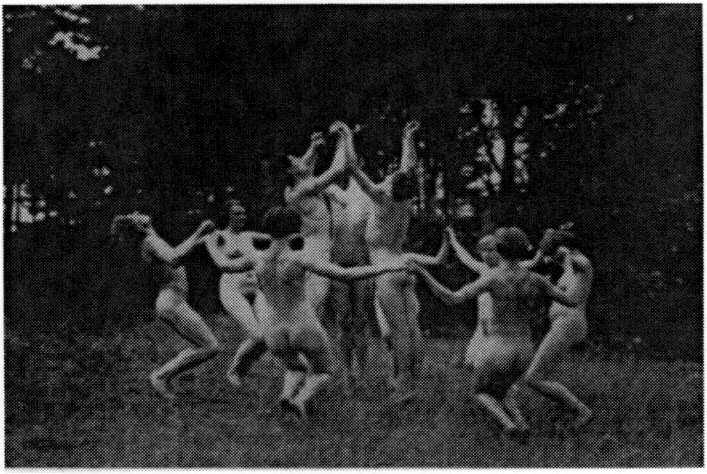

"Nudity and Education" which, having just been held in Berlin by Professor Koch, was the occasion for the article we found reprinted.

Elsewhere we discovered a circular announcement of this first "Congress" of free physical culture—November 23 to 25, 1929—of which Koch was the organizer. The program read as follows:

NUDITY AND EDUCATION

First Congress of the Adolf Koch School of Free Physical Culture (with the collaboration of the *Freikörperkultursparte* of Berlin-Brandenburg).

Saturday:

Reception of guests in the Koch School, with presentation of nude gymnastics.

Evening—Public meeting, "Why return to Nudity?"

Sunday:

Morning—Theatrical gymnastic performance.

Evening—Lectures by Clara Bohm-Schuch, Dr. Kawcrau, and Dr. Friedrich Wolf.

Monday:

Morning—Demonstration of the benefits of gymnastics.

Evening—Presentation of moving picture film, "New Ways in Gymnastics." Comments on film by Adolf Koch and Dr. Hans Graaz.

On Tuesday guests may witness the practical exercises of the Koch School.

. . . .

200 guests from outside Berlin, if members of the Koch Schools or of the *Volksgesundheit* group, will find free board and lodging at the homes of the Berlin friends, so that the total cost to them will be only that of their actual travelling expenses.

As to the success of this "Congress" we gained some inkling also from the pamphlet given us by Fräulein Adrian, for along with the extended account quoted from the *Vorwärts* were numerous other reports reprinted from German journals of practically every shade of opinion. Nearly all of them reviewed the Congress favourably.

From them we gleaned the facts that the meetings were attended by approximately 3000 people, of whom about 100 were official delegates from either socialist or bourgeois *Freikörperkultur* organizations in various sections of Germany. Twenty-five registered from foreign countries, including Argentina, Austria, Belgium, Czecho-Slovakia, France, Hungary, Poland, Russia, Switzerland—and the United States.

For there was a doctor from New York. Apparently *Nacktkultur* is not utterly unknown to all of America.

FRANCE

XII

FRENCH NUDISTS AND NATURISTS

When we left Germany for France, it was with the fear that were were leaving free-light bathing behind. Of course we had made inquiries from our German friends about the French movement and had been surprised to learn that there was one. But we were told—and this did not surprise us—that it was still small and rather timid in regard to practice.

An American tourist, judging the French mentality from Paris music halls, the books and postal cards displayed in certain shops around the Avenue de l'Opéra, and such periodicals as *La Vie Parisienne,* might think that France would be a fertile field for nudity. By this time, however, we had learned that nudity of *Nacktkultur* and the nudity —or, more strictly speaking, partial nudity—of pornography are utterly incompatible. It is illogical, but not astonishing, to find the Paris police permitting pornographic journals and books to be freely exhibited, while forbidding the display in the kiosks of a serious nudist review, and allowing the undress of the *Folies Bergère* while refusing to authorize a nudist sport field.

Anyone acquainted with French family life and bourgeois morality realizes that the idea of nudity in common would be as shocking to the French as to the Anglo-Saxons. In this one respect, French modesty goes even further perhaps than ours. One might assume that with the greater frankness of speech in France in regard to sexual matters and physical functions, both in literature and in the conversation of good society, the French would be more open-minded on the subject than Americans. It must not be forgotten, however, that in France a great gulf exists between the frankness of adult society on sexual questions and the education of children and young people.

The training of French children is even more prudish than that of our own. Co-education is virtually unknown in elementary and secondary schools. There is also a more clearly defined line between what is suitable for the young, particularly the young girl, and for the adult. Well brought up French girls are generally allowed much less freedom in reading matter than the average American girl. "Not suitable for the *jeune fille*" and "not to be put in all hands" are frequent comments on literature—even in the publishers' advertisements.

In America sexual education or hygiene for the young is coming to be recognized as a necessity, and many schools give such instruction, but in France instruction in these matters is for the most part still regarded as scandalous. The boy is left to pick up his knowledge from his comrades at school, and the girl to get along without any knowledge at all if she leads the sheltered life that prevails even today in many bourgeois families, in spite of the shaking-up of the war, with its resulting greater freedom for women.

Another cause for the difficulty with which nudist doctrines make headway in France is that physical culture has been adopted more recently and less widely in France than in the northern countries. Sports in late years have made much progress, but chiefly in the wealthy classes, where they are often a question of what the French call "*snobisme*." The schools are still without physical culture or organized athletics. Indeed, with the heavy program of the French *lycée*, the school boy or girl has almost no time for games or exercise even outside of school hours.

As for hygiene, it is well known that in France the daily tub or shower bath is still a luxury that has not penetrated to the lower classes, and that is out of the question even for many middle class families living in old apartment houses. The majority of the French sleep with closed windows and fear a draft far more than germs, as the tourist is well aware who has tried to keep a train window open in a compartment of French people. An intelligent Frenchwoman once said to us, "It seems that drafts are quite harmless in America, but here they are very dangerous. It must be the difference in the climate."

Whatever the reasons, the cult of nudity in France has to break down a deep-seated prejudice, a prudishness similar to what we have come to associate with the words "Anglo-Saxon."

It is significant that when the United States authorities a few years ago required the crews of incoming ships to undress for the medical examination at Quarantine, the first protest came from the French. The crew of the S.S. "Paris," rather than submit to this indignity, relinquished the privilege of going ashore while the ship was docked in New York, and the French Line complained through diplomatic channels of the disgrace that respectable seamen, "many of them fathers of families," should be forced to exhibit themselves naked.

It was also the French, characteristically enough, who protested recently to the Postal Union about the nude picture on the Spanish stamp commemorating the Goya Centennial —a reproduction of Goya's painting of the Duchess of Alva.

In Klingberg we had become acquainted with the magazines of the two French societies for free physical culture. *La Vie Sage,* which on May 1, 1930, changed its title to *Naturisme* and began to appear weekly instead of twice a month, is the organ of the *Société Naturiste* directed by the Doctors André and Gaston Durville. This society possesses a naturist centre with a large athletic field on the Island of Médan at Villennes-sur-Seine, not far from St. Germain-en-Laye. Here also they are constructing "Physiopolis," a bungalow colony where the members of the society may camp. The society is flourishing, and on week-ends the island is crowded, but—

The members of the *Société Naturiste* are not out-and-out nudists. They primarily advocate hygienic living conditions, a diet based on vegetarian principles, and exercises in the air and sunshine—in short, the preservation of health through natural means rather than a recourse to drugs and surgery. Total nudity, they admit, would be the ideal for sports and sunbathing, but they do not believe it practicable in France at the present time. Hence they have compromised. The minimum costume permitted at Villennes consists of trunks, which may be reduced to a mere triangle of cloth in front and behind, leaving the thighs completely bare, with the addition, in the case of women, of a brassière.

Less than this is not permitted, but there is no regulation costume; any sort of sport dress or semi-undress goes. The costumes are frequently impractical and sometimes ridiculous. The photographs in *Naturisme* of the games and exercises at Villennes lack the harmony of those of the real nudists. Some of the naturists wear tunics, others ample trunks, some bathing suits, and some the minimum costume —but even that in all colours, shapes and designs. Of course the free play of muscles in movement is missing in these pictures. The more ample costumes break the graceful lines of the bodies, while the scantiest costumes give, as one Frenchwoman said, "a music hall effect" and stress the very portions of the body they are designed to hide.

As the result of this compliance with convention, Villennes is the only *authorized* airbathing centre in the vicinity of Paris. In justice to the *Société Naturiste* we must say that they have had to choose between the sacrifice of complete nudity and that of their field at Villennes. At any rate, when the centre was started, the intention was to create a field where total nudity could be practised. The Durvilles petitioned the Prefect of Police for permission to do so, but conversations with officials in that department, as well as in the Ministry of the Interior, convinced the naturists that the authorities were resolved to prevent the practice of nudity, and to do it, as the Durvilles said, "by any means, legal or illegal."

Hence a year ago, *La Vie Sage,* while printing nude pictures, announced that costumes would be necessary at Villennes *temporarily.* Today, the naturists in the illustrations wear at least a loin cloth, and *La Vie Sage* in its last number under the old title declared in italics that *nobody had ever been naked* on the island.

The *Société Naturiste* has its reward. Villennes is undisturbed and freely advertised; it is the only centre for air-bathing of which many French people have heard; and *Naturisme* can be displayed in the kiosks.

It was the bi-monthly periodical of the smaller but more daring society, however, that attracted us. *Vivre Intégralement,* the organ of the *Amis de Vivre,* under the direction of M.-K. de Mongeot, has the courage of its convictions. As a result, the police have forbidden its display in the kiosks, although it can be sold there and, illogically enough, can be exhibited in the windows of the bookstores.

Vivre Intégralement declares flatly that the *Amis de Vivre* are nudists first and foremost, as distinguished from naturists. In fact, while discussing and advocating a healthy diet and temperate living, they do not exact any adherence to vegetarianism, alcoholic abstinence and the like. For them, these are side issues, and too much insistence on such principles might alienate people who otherwise would be sympathetic to the nudist idea.

As M. de Mongeot has stated in *Vivre,* "We are not gymnosophists, and still less gymnomystics; we are merely men of our epoch who seek to re-establish by means of health the equilibrium between the soul and the body. We are far from having the idea that a return to nature is a panacea; we take from it only the benefits it offers us, as we reject of civilization and progress only what is harmful to our well-being."

Vivre, like the German reviews, publishes photographs of men, women and children as God made them. This was encouraging. But we could not discover from its columns that they had any permanent centre for practising nudity. There were reports from Algiers, Marseilles and a few other provincial cities indicating that groups of members there made excursions on Sundays. Deep mystery, however, surrounded the activity of the Paris group. Herr Zimmermann had told us that during the previous summer the Paris group had met on Sundays at a country estate, but he did not know whether they still had the place. To be sure, in a back number of *Vivre* we found a cryptic notice:

> THE GYMNASTIC CLUB
>
> will be open in May in a pleasant and healthy country region, an hour and a half from Paris.
> It is possible to stay there from Saturday to Monday.
> *Amis de Vivre,* inquire immediately about terms for membership.

What was the Gymnastic Club? There was nothing to indicate whether their sessions were held in "integral nudity" or not. Was it officially connected with *Vivre?* As the notice was set off in a box, it might be nothing more than an advertisement of an entirely separate organization.

Monsieur de Mongeot, however, seemed to be the person most capable of aiding us in our quest for French nudists. No sooner did we arrive in Paris than we sought him out in the offices of *Vivre,* near the Parc Monceau.

The offices are in a small building that serves for both publishing house and gymnasium; in the same building is held the physical culture course of Monsieur Gilbert de Mongeot, equipped with ultra-violet lamps for heliotherapy. The little hallway that we entered from the street is traversed constantly by men in track suits and by messengers from bookstores who carry away packages of paper-bound volumes. In addition to its magazine, *Vivre* from time to time publishes de luxe brochures on various aspects of the theory and practice of nudity and a number of books on such subjects as heliotherapy. They also keep in stock for sale a large number of books on physical culture, naturism, hygiene and the like. Some of the works of Havelock Ellis and H. G. Wells, in French translations, are among the volumes they handle.

We made known our errand to a young man in trunks, who called Monsieur de Mongeot. The director of the *Amis de Vivre* is young, tall and robust, with curling blond hair and blue eyes. He looks Scandinavian rather than Latin, and his manner is reserved and totally lacking in the vivacity one expects from the French. The long white smock he wore gave him a surgical appearance, heightening the impression of coolness and calm.

His welcome to us was cordial, however; he escorted us into his tiny office, and to our surprise lit a cigarette. Evidently the nudist leaders in France are not so convinced of the harmfulness of tobacco as they are of that of clothing.

There was, he told us, no permanent nudist camp in France, but the *Amis de Vivre* did have a centre outside of Paris where they went for week-ends, and where they were arranging rooms for members of the society who wished to spend their vacations in the park. Camping facilities were already available. He cordially invited us to come to the meeting the following Sunday.

"You can take the eight o'clock train for Choseville.[1] Someone will meet you at the station. Bring your lunch so that you can spend the whole day inside the park."

"But that is rather far from Paris, is it not?" we asked. "The distance must keep away many people who would like to come—at least keep them from coming as often as they might to a more accessible place. The rail fare alone is no small item."

"It is unfortunate," agreed Monsieur de Mongeot, "but what do you wish? Any nearer to Paris, we should be sure to have trouble. We have to be in a remote and quiet district."

"The people of Choseville then are indifferent?"

"They know nothing about it. If the attention of the municipality were drawn to our centre, we should no doubt have difficulty. We have a private estate and the country people have no idea of what goes on inside the walls."

"You own the estate?"

[1] For the protection of our French nudist friends, we must preserve the anonymity of their centre. This is the only place in which we have used fictitious geographic names.

"We rent it," he replied. "The owner knows what the property is used for, but that is all. This is the second summer we have had the place, and no one has displayed any curiosity."

We asked him then whether there were branches of *Vivre* in the provinces that practised the nudist doctrines regularly.

"Yes, we have active groups in Marseilles, Algiers, Lyons and Strasbourg in France, as well as in Belgium. Groups are being formed in Bordeaux, Toulon and Nice. Here are some photographs of the Algerian and Marseillais groups."

On the white sands of a North African beach, French men, women and children were playing games or basking in the sun. The Provençal friends of *Vivre* were clambering among rocks overhanging the Mediterranean, or forming antique friezes against a background of huge classic columns.

"The Marseilles group is very fortunate," Monsieur de Mongeot explained. "Not only is their centre authorized by the municipality, but the city government has given them the use of an island, the Ile Frioul, where there is an old *lazaret,* or quarantine station for ships entering the harbour."

"How does it happen that the municipality of Marseilles is so much more tolerant than that of Paris, for instance?"

"M. Sabiani, the deputy-mayor, is interested in our movement."

"How many members are there in the *Amis de Vivre?*" we inquired.

"About two thousand—not many compared with the nudists in Germany—but the society is only two years old. The Marseilles group alone has over eighty members. *Vivre Intégralement* is in its fifth year, but we believed it necessary first to advocate the idea and accustom people to it, before attempting to form centres for putting our doctrines into practise."

"What do you find is the chief obstacle to your progress in France? Obstruction from the public powers? The interference of moralists?"

"Ridicule!" was the prompt reply. "The French spirit of mockery. Our adversaries paint comic pictures of Tardieu or Briand speaking in the Chamber of Deputies in the costume of Adam, of Monsieur Doumic presiding over a session of naked Academicians. They don't bother to find out that we do not advocate the immediate discarding of all clothes on all occasions, that the only costume we war against is the sport costume. The public laughs and refuses to take nudism seriously."

Although French wit is undoubtedly one of the greatest obstacles encountered by nudist propaganda in France, there is legal interference, as the ordinance forbidding the display of *Vivre* demonstrates. Even now a case is pending which may lead to nudist doctrines being discussed for the first time in the Palace of Justice. The *Fédération Française des Sociétés contre l'Immoralité* has brought suit against Dr. Pierre Vachet, Professor in the School of Psychology, and M. de Mongeot for the publication by the *Editions de Vivre* in 1928 of Dr. Vachet's book on *La Nudité et la Physiologie Sexuelle.*

Anyone familiar with the scientific nature of Dr. Vachet's works might believe that the French Anti-Immorality Societies could find better examples of the dissemination of vicious and obscene literature in France. But censorship and societies for the suppression of vice frequently suffer from a strange "pornography-blindness." Monsieur de Mongeot is inclined to think that the animosity of the *Fédération Française* toward Dr. Vachet is religious in origin, and that Vachet's real offence was the publication of a book on the miracles of Lourdes.[1]

A few more questions, and we thanked Monsieur de Mongeot for his information, promising to be at Choseville on Sunday morning. Indeed we were more than eager to go, in order to compare the French practice of nudity with that in Germany. The reactions of two peoples so different in temperament and mentality ought to give us a fair basis for judging the adaptability of free physical culture to various peoples and civilizations.

One of the common arguments of opponents to nudism outside of Germany is founded on national differences. Nudity is a German invention, suited to the character and intellect of Germanic races, they say, but totally unfitted for other peoples—Latins or Anglo-Saxons, for instance. We should see for ourselves how Latins take to nudist doctrines.

[1] Since this was written, the case has been dismissed for lack of grounds.

XIII

A CHÂTEAU IN NORMANDY

SUNDAY DAWNED CLEAR FOR OUR EXPEDITION TO THE park of the Paris nudists. We set out for Normandy, armed with a package containing a lunch—not strictly vegetarian. Indeed, if Paris hotel dwellers tried to assemble a vegetarian meal from the nearest *charcuteries,* they would find themselves limited to fruit and olives, scarcely filling after a morning of exercise in the open air.

We had about an hour and a half on the train and, as on the way to Gleschendorf, we attempted to pick out nudists among our fellow travellers. The three supernaturally quiet and well-behaved little girls, under the convoy of a sturdy peasant *nounou,* scarcely looked as if they were bound for a romp in a "Free-Light Park." They were much too pale and subdued. While their nurse dozed in the corner, they sat, little gloved hands sedately folded in their laps, as motionless as small idols, and during the whole trip ventured only a few whispered comments to each other.

It was even more unlikely that the other occupant of our compartment was a nudist. He was a white-haired, white-moustached man of seventy or more, lean, but with the protruding belly of an inactive old age. He was wearing an unusual variety of decorations, a ribbon and a rosette in his coat lapel, and an entirely different ribbon and rosette in the buttonhole of his overcoat. Probably a retired army officer leading a sedentary life, whose chief diversion was an *apéritif* and a game of piquet in some favourite café.

He took from his pocket a morning edition of *L'Ami du Peuple* and settled down to read it. *L'Ami du Peuple* is the latest creation of M. François Coty, the celebrated perfumer, and is conservative, nationalistic, and militaristic in the extreme.

"Well," said Mason, "that settles it. He's no nudist. He hasn't had a new idea since 1870."

At Choseville the corridors were crowded with what seemed an unusually large number of people to be getting off at a town of its size and importance. Perhaps there were some nudists on the train after all.

Outside the station exit, we looked for our guide. But M. de Mongeot was not there, we could see nothing resembling an official reception committee, and we did not know a single French nudist by sight except the director. We did not even know the name of the estate where we were going, or how far it was from Choseville. We began to feel somewhat lost. Would it do, we speculated, to approach any of the travellers coming from the station with the question, "*Pardon, monsieur, êtes-vous nudiste?*"

A number of people were gathering in front of the station,

evidently preparing to get into a large bus. But surely they were not the ones we were seeking; they were too unlike our conception of nudists, the hardy gymnasts with whom we had become acquainted in Germany. The women were elegantly dressed, with the high heels and the rouged lips of the Parisienne; the men also looked as if they would be more at home on the Boulevards than on the athletic field.

Then our eyes fell on a man who might at least lead an outdoor life. Bareheaded and sunburned, he wore a soft shirt, open at the neck, and carried a knapsack on his back. With him was a tanned lad of about ten. We approached this healthy looking gentleman and tentatively murmured the name of Monsieur de Mongeot.

"Ah, you are going to the Château de Machin too? Let me see, there is the bus and a couple of other cars, but I am afraid they are full. I am walking with some of the others."

"How far is it?" we asked.

"About seven kilometres."

We were taken aback, not so much at the idea of walking so far as at the thought of wasting so much precious time outside the gates of the French paradise. But a rescuing angel suddenly appeared beside us in the person of a well-dressed man in his late thirties.

"Will you come with us?" he asked, waving his hand toward a new sedan parked in the station square.

We accepted thankfully, and he introduced his wife, a charming and gracious young woman.

Monsieur and Madame Régnier had driven from Paris that morning—we learned from their card that they lived on a fashionable street near the Bois de Boulogne—but because they had never been to the Château de Machin, they had waited for the train at Choseville to get instructions about the road.

But the instructions proved to be of little avail. The streets of Choseville are a picturesque labyrinth from which it is difficult to emerge—at least on the right road. Decidedly the sunbathing park is not well known in the neighbourhood. Most of the townsmen of Choseville had never heard of the Château de Machin. At last, however, after making several experimental sallies into the country, M. Régnier found a road that some peasants assured him would take us there.

"We are going to see how we like it," explained Madame Régnier. "If we do, we shall bring our children next Sunday."

M. Régnier was astonished that we had discovered *Vivre* and the Château de Machin.

"Many French people have never heard of it," he said, "especially now that *Vivre* is not on display in the kiosks. It is only recently that I learned about the movement myself and went to see Monsieur de Mongeot."

"My husband," interrupted Madame Régnier, "has always liked to be in the sun and air without clothes. Whenever he finds a secluded corner of a garden, he undresses. But I've never done such a thing. I don't know whether I shall have the courage before all these people. Perhaps when everybody else is like that, it won't be so hard."

We attempted to encourage her with accounts of our own recent initiation.

A Château in Normandy

The Château de Machin was reached finally, though the road, instead of approaching the entrance, skirted a long extent of high wall, for the park, unlike the *Freilichtpark* at Klingberg, is impenetrably screened and fortified. In fact, it looked for a time as if there were no entrance, and Madame Régnier, whose terror was visibly increasing, might have ordered a retreat if the rest of us had not been so eager to storm the fort.

Eventually, by driving across a meadow, we discovered the way in, on quite another road from the one we had taken, and we halted at the gate of the Château. The bus, although having left Choseville after us, was already there, and the first person we saw on the lawn, hobbling along stiffly with a cane, was the retired military man of *L'Ami du Peuple!* Never again will we venture to identify nudists at sight.

M. de Mongeot, draped majestically in a dressing gown and shod in sandals, received us. With him, also in dressing gown, was Madame de Mongeot, as French—dark and vivacious—as he is un-French. We were shown the Château, a fine old house that has suffered from neglect, but that was being put into order as a *pension* for the *Amis de Vivre*. Since the Château and its lawn are open to the highway, nudity, as at Klingberg, is permitted only within the park, which is entered by a gate close to the house.

Inside the densely wooded park is a small hunting lodge used for dressing rooms—gentlemen downstairs and ladies above. Before it, in a sunny clearing, half a dozen naked men, and a young woman in a bathing suit, were playing ball. Did the French women, after all, lack the courage of the women across the Rhine? We inquired of Madame de

Mongeot, who had guided us, still wrapped in her dressing gown.

"Oh, no," she explained, "that young woman is wearing a bathing suit only because the morning air is a little chilly."

"Are there any other women here, undressed?" asked Madame Régnier apprehensively.

"But yes. There are a number in different parts of the woods. As the park contains fifteen hectares (between 35 and 40 acres), it is easy to lose the others. But we shall find several young girls at the playground."

"Young girls, really?" Madame Régnier was astounded. "When I was a young girl, I should never have dared to do such a thing."

As we started into the dressing room, Madame Régnier appealed desperately to Madame de Mongeot: "May I wear a bathing suit, *madame?* I brought one."

"Since it is your first time, yes. I have one on under my dressing gown. I shall keep it on, too, if you prefer."

Here Frances intervened with no less desperation than Madame Régnier:

"But I have no bathing suit. Please, somebody keep me company. I haven't the courage to be the only naked lady, and I certainly don't want to remain completely dressed."

"Very well," said Madame Régnier bravely, "I shall undress *intégralement*. After all, nobody here knows me."

When we came from the dressing rooms—Madame Régnier shrinking but urged on by her husband—we ran through the woods to the clearing used for games.

The park at Machin is in a wilder state of nature than that at Klingberg. The paths strewn with stones and twigs demand shoes or sandals, and the open space used for sports has only recently been cleared of brush. There are still treacherous tree stubs protruding from the earth. The rolling and writhing on the ground required by some of exercises we had practised in Germany would be out of the question here.

Nevertheless we found thirty or forty gymnasts assembled, including several children and the elderly reader of *L'Ami du Peuple*. A fair-haired boy of three, evidently a neophyte, was weeping bitterly because his mother was removing his bathing suit, but in a few minutes he was romping like a puppy with two little girls and the boy we had seen at the station. The aspect of the group, aside from the slighter build of the French physique, differed from that of a group in a German *Nacktkultur* park only in the smaller proportion of women.

Under the leadership of a young man we went through a series of vigorous setting-up exercises. The old man of *L'Ami du Peuple* abandoned his cane and strove valiantly to keep up with the rest, sketching abortive gestures with his decrepit limbs, at once pathetic and grotesque. Ball games followed, the same games as in Germany, and then lunch on the grass in front of the hunting lodge.

Another difference between German and French nudists was at once apparent: the latter are more afraid of taking cold. The hardiest lunched without clothing, but many, although the air was warm, slipped on bathing suits, coats or sweaters. The old man donned a flannel undershirt.

During lunch we had a better opportunity to make the acquaintance of the group. Monsieur de Mongeot had already told us that most of the *Amis de Vivre* were of the intellectual and professional classes, many of them teachers or physicians.

Among the doctors who are members are Dr. Chauvet, laureate of the Faculty and Hospitals of Paris, Dr. Dausset, head of a department of the Hôtel-Dieu, Dr. Charles Guilbert, head of a hospital laboratory, Professor Laignet-Lavastine, of the Paris hospitals, Dr. Legrain, who has many official titles including that of Medical Expert for the Courts and Military Boards of the Seine, Dr. de Marville, former head surgeon of the French Hospital in San Francisco, and Dr. Pierre Vachet, Professor in the School of Psychology.

Professor Charles Richet of the Institute of France, and Professor Pierre Pruvost of the University of Lille are prominent scholars who endorse the movement. Journalism has a distinguished representative in Maurice de Waleffe, editor-in-chief of *Paris-Midi,* who has wittily defended the nudists in the public press. Lieutenant-General Kestens, Minister of National Defence in Belgium during the war, and Commandant Yves Le Prieur of the Naval Academy represent the professional warriors. The titled aristocracy has a couple of *Marquis* on *Vivre's* list and His Indian Highness the Prince of Kapurthala.

Though none of these "personalities" were disporting themselves at the Château de Machin the Sunday of our visit, we found about sixty people of every age, type and condition. There were professional men, an artist who sketched some of the groups lunching on the grass, well-to-do people

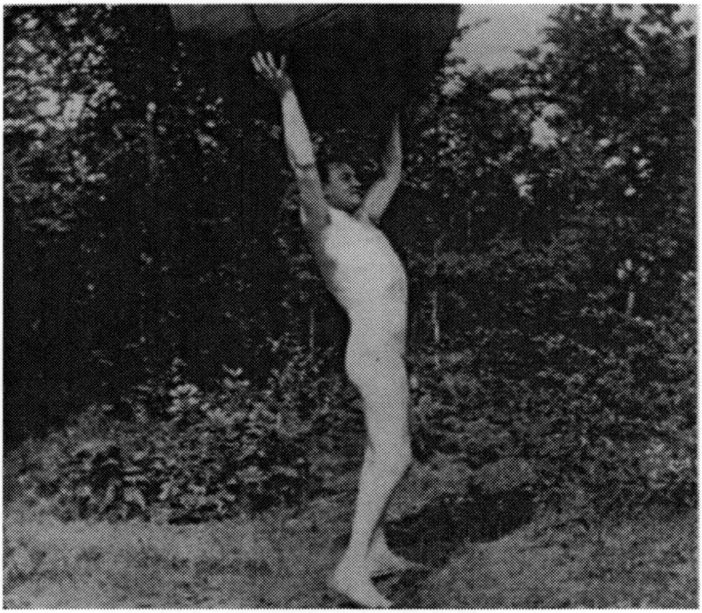

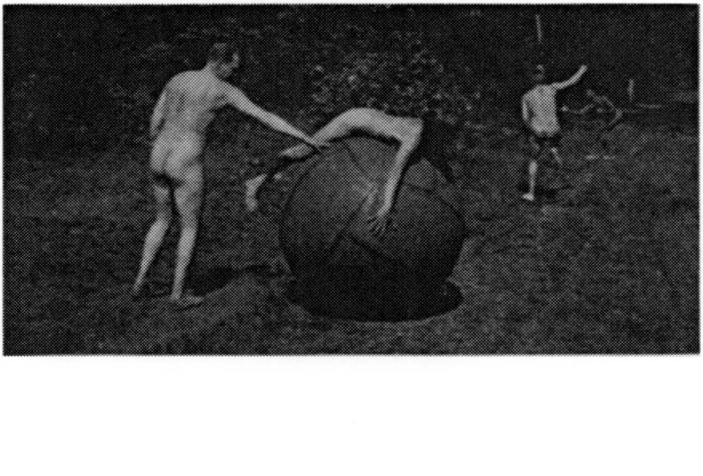

of the upper middle class, *petits bourgeois,* a sea captain and a chef. There were bronzed athletic young men, a few girls with slender lithe bodies, portly middle-aged business men, and plump matrons. The man to whom we had first spoken at the Choseville station—the one who looked as if he led an outdoor life—proved to be the sea captain.

A frail appearing war *mutilé* who had acquired an uncanny skill at games and physical labour with his left arm, was accompanied by his healthy wife and two small girls, as brown as little gypsies. This family of thorough-going naturists ate a strictly vegetarian luncheon, the main dish of which was a salad of mixed vegetables.

Among the crowd we found only one other foreigner besides ourselves—another difference, for the group at Klingberg was much more international. He was an Englishman, a continental agent for a big transatlantic steamship line. We wondered whether he would bring his influence to bear on the company for the installation of nudist sun decks—"nudariums"—on its liners.

We were shocked to discover, seated on a canvas garden chair among the picnickers, the indecent spectacle of a lady whose age the French would call "certain" and we "uncertain," fully clad, with a newspaper over her head as protection from the sun's rays.

"Why doesn't your wife undress?" someone asked her husband, a mature but well-preserved gentleman who, "practising" the integral life for the first time, had expanded in the sun like a plant. We had observed the delight and abandon with which he had frolicked all the forenoon.

He shrugged his shoulders with cheerful resignation: "She

says she hasn't the proper shoes, and it's my fault of course because I didn't tell her to bring sandals. But one does not argue with the ladies."

Madame's high-heeled slippers were indeed unsuitable for romping through the paths of the Château de Machin, but perhaps a more powerful deterrent was the fact that she was older and fatter than most of the other women. The sour expression with which she watched the nudists indicated that she considered the whole business stuff and nonsense. But if her spouse would go to such places, then *grand dieu!* she would go too and keep an eye on him.

During lunch, the nudists around us talked of travel, summer resorts, and, naturally, the movement and its centres. Some of those present had been to Villennes, the naturist island in the Seine, but they had found it too crowded and the costumes ridiculous. One man who had spent much time in Belgium said that the movement there was small; Belgium was too "black." A couple of people who had lived in Spain agreed that it would be difficult for the movement to make progress in that country, where women are still comparatively unemancipated.

They discussed the reasons that make it harder for a woman to bring herself to appearing unclothed in public, agreeing that the most potent were vanity and the education which inculcates what the Victorians called "female modesty." One lady remarked, "Women are afraid to come, but they lose their fear the first time—as soon as they have seen that the other women are ugly too."

This, by the way, is an answer to the objection sometimes made that the illustrations of the nudist reviews are inartistic since they show old and misshapen bodies as well as the graceful, well-proportioned forms of beautiful youth. These pictures revealing the human figure as it actually is, with all the defects that centuries of unhygienic living and clothing have inflicted on the majority of us, are more encouraging to men and women conscious of their own physical imperfections than the lovely, harmonious bodies that answer all the requirements of classical art.

In one respect the conversation of the nudists was remarkable to anyone familiar with the customary freedom of French wit in even the most correct circles. There were none of the spicy jests, the risqué innuendoes of the *esprit gaulois*. Madame Régnier, increasingly delighted with her new experience, was the first to call our attention to the fact that the talk was more proper than in a salon, despite a gaiety and animation that often reached the point of hilarity. For there was nothing stiff or solemn about the decorum of the nudists.

After lunch we rested on the grass in the sun, and then gradually the crowd dispersed, some groups wandering through the grounds, others resuming ball games, and the laziest merely chatting and basking in the sun. We took the opportunity to ask Monsieur de Mongeot further questions about the *Amis de Vivre,* and he gave us the printed regulations governing the park of Machin, with the application blank for membership in the club.

The questionnaire on the application blank was similar to that which must be filled out when requesting the use of the Klingberg *Freilichtpark,* except for the requirement —significant of woman's status in France—that the application of a woman must be accompanied by the authorization of her husband. As for the rules, most of them were word for word the same as those at Klingberg. In fact, Herr Zimmermann had given his rules to Monsieur de Mongeot, who translated a number of them.

The distinctive feature of the regulations of the French club is the preamble, which is worth reproducing as an apt and sincere statement of the aims of the French organization:

> "Our end is to develop the individual wholly and harmoniously, employing the natural elements fitted for maintaining the proper balance of his being, and making him evolve toward the beautiful and good. We adopt the Greek ideal *kalos kagathos*, the beautiful and good man, persuaded that by making efforts to attain this end we shall contribute to the amelioration of humanity and a better mutual understanding among mankind—consequently to a fraternity of peoples, without weakness, and indispensable for the exchange of customs, industries, arts and sciences.
>
> "We believe that the love of humanity is tributary to the love of one's country.
>
> "Our ideal is compatible with that of all religions and may become that of unbelievers."

When Monsieur de Mongeot was called away—the director was constantly in demand by members seeking information or wishing to discuss proposed improvements at Machin—we explored the grounds.

The park had evidently been laid out years before with walks or shaded *allées* after the formal fashion of the gardens designed by Le Nôtre. Still radiating from circular lawns, where tall, wild grass was surrounded by crumbling benches, were faint, overgrown paths, their geometric pattern nearly obliterated. Along them we raced, delighted once more to run in the woods, with the feel of the wind on our bare bodies.

But all too soon it was time to think of the six o'clock train from Choseville and the habiliments of the outer world. There was a joyous splashing and shrieking around the well as we took showers by the primitive process of throwing water on one another, or soused ourselves in the big tub under the pump. The chief drawback to the Château de Machin at the present time is the lack of bathing facilities, but they are planning to install an outdoor shower and clean out a little pond in the park—now stagnant and uninviting —for a swimming pool.

There was great merriment when one of the ladies strayed by accident into the gentlemen's dressing room. *Quel scandale!*

"I was shocked," she announced. "They were in suspenders—too ugly by far."

Madame Régnier resumed her clothing with as much reluctance as she had taken it off.

"How uncomfortable it is," she sighed, "with all these stupid things that women wear, corsets and brassières."

"And the stupid things that men wear, stiff collars and garters and suspenders," added her husband.

"Are you bringing your children next Sunday?" we asked.

"Certainly," was the reply. "We are sorry we did not have them with us today."

"One thing worries me though," confessed Madame Régnier. "I'm afraid they will tell my parents. Our little girl is so talkative. My people would be horribly shocked, for they are very conservative. We told them we were going picnicking with friends today."

"We shall make the children promise not to tell," interposed Monsieur Régnier, "or we shan't bring them again. They'll have such a good time that they will be crazy to come back."

It was with sincere regret that we took leave of the *Amis de Vivre* and their château in Normandy, with real sorrow in fact, for it was a sort of farewell to free physical culture itself. In a few days—before the next Sunday—we had embarked at Hâvre for America.

THE MOVEMENT IN GENERAL

XIV

THE SPREAD OF NUDISM IN EUROPE

DOUBTLESS FEW AMERICANS HAVE ANY MORE OF AN idea than we had before our trip to Europe of the extent of the nudist movement and the serious attention it is attracting abroad. Certainly our experience since we returned to this country would indicate a lack of any general knowledge or comprehension of it on the part of our countrymen.

Even in New York, in the so-called intellectual class, which theoretically should be best informed regarding ideas and events in Europe, we have found nothing more than a vague notion that a few foreign freaks and fanatics have sporadic outbursts of trying to live without clothes, manifesting either a scandalous libertinism or a hare-brained back-to-naturism. If Americans have heard of nudist colonies, they have put them down at best as aggregations of cranks, the zealots of a mad Utopia, no more significant or interesting, save in their shocking aspects, than the colony of some crazy prophet of a new religious or social scheme.

Yet American ignorance and incredulity on the subject are understandable when one observes the sort of notice the European manifestations receive in our daily press. American newspapers have published few accurate accounts that attempt to give a clear explanation of the background and significance of the incidents featured.

There was one good story in the New York *Times* for July 13, 1930, on the naturist colony at Villennes-sur-Seine. The writer, P. J. Philip, not only described the island and the people who frequent it, but he gave an intelligent exposition of their creed and aims. However, the *Naturistes* not being nudists, strictly speaking, this can scarcely be considered even one of the exceptions that prove the rule.

Another story in the New York *Evening World,* for last August 21, gave an accurate and extended account of the spread of the movement in Germany. It contained, nevertheless, a typically preposterous statement regarding nudist activities in France, which included, according to the correspondent, a nude march in the principal streets of Paris.

Usually the best items shown to us upon our return to this country have been nothing more than bare statements of facts, possibly true, such as the Associated Press dispatch from San Sebastian, Spain, in the New York *World* for July 12, 1930. Three sentences made the entire story: "Bathers in certain portions of Concha Beach will hereafter be permitted to take sunbaths in natural suits. Up to the present the police have arrested bathers who forgot to cover themselves. Now, however, sun fadists will be allowed to go about as they desire."

Generally, however, the newspaper story is an absurd yarn, resembling the one in a Texas paper which stated that Paris dressmakers were being bankrupted by the spread of the naturist movement started by the Doctors Durville, and that Parisiennes no longer wore dresses but were going naked! And a summer or two ago there was a widely printed story to the effect that the Berlin police had arrested thousands of *Lichtfreunde* who insisted on strolling in the city parks during the hot weather attired only in their skins.

This tale caused much merriment among the German nudist leaders to whom the clipping had been sent. Probably the Berlin police would have acted about as was reported if the circumstances had arisen, but the nudists would undoubtedly have known better than to attempt such a wholesale and revolutionary demonstration.

Typical of the imaginative exaggerations of our foreign correspondents is a story that appeared in the New York *Evening World* on June 28, 1930. In the column "World's Window," Pierre Van Paassen, giving a sprightly account of Paris news, wrote:

"The nudist colony of Paris has addressed a letter to the Prefect of Police asking his permission to extend their activities to the city itself. Hitherto they walked around 'in naturalibus' on a discreet little island in the Seine. This is not enough. . . . It's not likely in spite of the moving appeal on behalf of the pores that the Prefect will grant the request. Even a Prefect of Police must take into account the slow evolution of fashion."

Having this called to our attention when we were fresh from our investigation of the French nudist movement, we could easily pick the flaws in the story, which certainly gave the impression that the French nudists are completely lacking in common sense, if not sanity.

In the first place, "the nudist colony of Paris" is vague. There is only one out-and-out nudist society in Paris, to be sure—the *Amis de Vivre*—but the "discreet little island in the Seine" referred to in the second sentence belongs, not to it, but to the *Société Naturiste,* who are primarily naturists, as their name implies, and not nudists. As we have already stated in the account of our French experiences, the *Naturistes* have never "walked around *in naturalibus*" on their island.

Secondly, when they petitioned the Prefect of Police a year ago for permission to have a field for nude sunbathing on a part of their island, the response was of a nature to make the society abandon the idea and ever since call attention publicly and repeatedly to the fact that costumes are, and always have been, absolutely essential on the Ile de Villennes. It is highly unlikely that the *Naturistes* would even dare to hope Prefect Chiappe would be more lenient about the Paris streets than about an enclosed corner of a private island.

And it is also improbable that this was just a little joke of theirs, for they have displayed the greatest care to conciliate the authorities. The police are not noted for their sense of humour, and a joke even in France runs the danger of being taken seriously by certain reformers, such as one Abbé Béthléem, who seems to be the contemporary French Anthony Comstock.

Of course, the correspondent may have been confused

about the island on the Seine, and have had in mind the *Amis de Vivre*. But when one knows Monsieur de Mongeot and the leaders of *Vivre,* the story is even more fantastic. The *Amis de Vivre* have never sought authorization for a nudist park even outside of Paris, for they are fully aware of the futility of trying to. Their policy is to achieve their ends through the dissemination of their ideas by serious propaganda without sensational publicity. Seeking the support of sane scientists and educators, they are not interested in exploding bombs under the Prefect of Police.

Moreover, they have never advocated, even theoretically, going nude on the city streets. Jokes about naked ladies and gentlemen in the *Metro* they regard as one of the most unjustified weapons used against them. To paraphrase Mr. Van Paassen, even nudists take into account the slow evolution of fashion.

Why these strange tales should be the chief publicity our press gives the European nudists, we would not venture to say. We suspect that in the not distant future more exact and definite information will percolate to the American public; but in the meantime it is hard for us to keep our sanity above suspicion when we talk of our recent experiences.

First of all we must persuade our friends of the proportions of the movement, and the fact that intelligent, even prominent, Europeans are taking it seriously.

The movement in Germany, unsuspected as it may be in the United States, has reached such proportions that to survey it in all its ramifications would require an extended investigation. The results would fill a volume. It is not possible even to find accurate statistics as to the number of *Lichtfreunde* in Germany. For there are many nudists who do not belong to any organization, but who practise their doctrines privately, either at home or in unfrequented spots in the country. In fact, most of the guests at Klingberg, as is the case of those in other public camps, are not enrolled in any of the nudist clubs or federations. The figures available include only the members of recognized *Bunds* or leagues, and are not entirely accurate even for them, since new *Bunds* or new branches of old ones are constantly being organized.

A newspaper story under a Berlin date line of last August 10, states that there are 3,000,000 Germans now practising nudity. One French writer gave 200,000 as the official count of the German *Lichtfreunde* two years ago, but he adds that this figure not only fails to include those who practise at home but omits those belonging to unfederated clubs, such as Robert Laurer's *Liga für freie Lebensgestaltung.* This is a serious omission because Laurer's *Liga,* one of the largest in Germany, is virtually a federation in itself, with sixteen fields scattered throughout the country, from Hamburg in the North to Munich in the South, and from Cologne on the Rhine to Koenigsberg in East Prussia.

In the Socialist-Labour groups practising *Nacktkultur,* according to figures given by Adolf Koch a few months ago in one of his publications, there are no less than 60,000 members. This includes a number of organizations (among them the Koch schools), such as the *Touristenverein Die Naturfreunde,* the *Arbeiter-Turn-und Sportbund* (with which is affiliated the *Freiluftbund* that we visited near Hamburg), the *Sozialistiche Arbeiterjugend,* and the *Turnverein Fichte.* The largest of the federations whose membership is not recruited from any one class is the *Reichsverband für Freikörperkultur,* generally known as the R F K. The May number of its official publication, *Freikörperkultur und Lebensreform,* lists eleven affiliated clubs in Berlin alone, where their membership is said to be over 5000. Outside of the Berlin-Brandenburg area, the federation is divided into seven districts as follows: Northeast (5 clubs, 2 of which are in Stettin); Northwest (10 clubs, 2 in Hannover); West Germany (7 clubs, 2 in Dortmund and 2 in Cologne); Southwest (6 clubs); Central Germany (11 clubs, 3 in Dresden, 2 in Leipzig, and 2 in Dessau); Silesia (the *Lichtbund Schlesien,* affiliated with the R F K, has a number of groups, and there are at least two other clubs in Breslau); Bavaria (13 clubs, 3 in Munich, 2 in Nürnberg).

There are probably few German cities of any importance without some kind of a *Nacktkultur* organization. Berlin is said to have no less than thirty such clubs. There are numerous fields or parks devoted to physical culture in total nudity on the lakes in its vicinity; those on the Motzensee and the Uedersee are the best known.

But the activities of the *Lichtfreunde* are not confined to the fields or gymnasiums belonging to these innumerable *Bunds.* One of their most remarkable enterprises is the *Lichtschule* of Dr. Fränzel, at Glüsingen in the Lüneburger Heide, a co-educational school for young children, where pupils and teachers practise total nudity. Dr. Fränzel's unique institution is officially recognized by the state and gives the regular program of the German secondary schools. Besides being a school, Glüsingen is a vacation colony similar to that of Klingberg, for Dr. Fränzel also takes adult boarders who wish to practise *Freikörperkultur* in his large park.

Another celebrated nudist colony not a part of the activities of any society is at Klappholttal, on the large Island of Sylt, in the North Sea. Nude bathing on the fine white beaches there is authorized by the government of Schleswig-Holstein.

Even more astonishing to Anglo-Saxons is the fact that two public swimming pools in Berlin, the *Stadtbad* and the fashionable *Lunabad*—a pool with artificial waves and a café-restaurant—are turned over at specified hours and days to the nudists. At *Lunabad* they frolic in the surf and drink coffee on the balcony in the dress of Eden. The only incongruous note is the waiter, who is fully clad. For Americans, such official authorization of *Nacktkultur*, its recognition by municipalities and the state, is the most extraordinary feature of the movement in Germany.

We in this country can perhaps comprehend how numbers of Germans might be convinced of the benefits of *Nacktkultur* and put their ideas into practise, but it is not so easy to accustom ourselves to the fact that *Nacktkultur* is open and respectable. With our background of censorship and prohibition, of hypocrisy and bootlegging, we cannot help feeling that nudism—no matter how convinced we may be of its morality—must be clandestine.

Whenever we describe the German nudist periodicals, with their illustrations devoid of fig leaves, our friends immediately ask: "But how do they sell such things? Surely they can't send them through the mails."

The number of these magazines in itself is impressive. *Schönheit* (founded in 1902), *Freikörperkultur und Lebensreform* (the organ of the R F K), *Licht-Land* and *Lachendes Leben* (published by Robert Laurer), *Freie Körperkultur in Wort und Bild* and *Volks-Gesundheit* (both issued by Adolf Koch), *Figaro, Pelagius, Soma,* and *Asa* are a few titles of the chief of these periodicals. The real wonder for us, however, is that they are displayed and mailed as openly as the *Literary Digest* and are bought by all classes of people.

A striking instance of the freedom from interference is the gymnastic exhibition that Adolf Koch staged in the *Volksbühne* theatre in Berlin in November 1929. Although the performers, young people of both sexes, were entirely nude, there was no censorship. The general press in fact reviewed the performance with praise both for its beauty and usefulness.

But it was not always so. Up to the time of the Republic, the activities of the nudist societies (there were as many as 300 of them in Germany on the eve of the war) were more or less surreptitious. But with the new government began a reign of tolerance. As long as the nudists confine their nudity to the special localities reserved to them, or to unfrequented spots, they do not have to reckon with the law or official censorship. In fact, the Ministry of Health supports the movement, not only for its hygienic value, but as a weapon against vice.

Yet the nudists still have to face opposition. Bitter campaigns have been waged against them by both individuals and private organizations. The new *Kultur,* naturally enough, is distasteful to the most conservative elements. Some of the conspicuous leaders of the movement have been persecuted, and in a few cases have suffered materially. There is the instance of a clergyman, Pastor Weidemann, whose activities in behalf of *Nacktkultur* led to his losing his church. And there is Hans Surén, an ex-army officer, whose book *Die Mensch und die Sonne* is one of the outstanding works on *Freikörperkultur.* When he applied his system of nude gymnastics to the training of the men under him, he was dismissed from the army. But others, such as Adolf Koch, have triumphed.

In attitude toward the movement, there is a marked difference between northern and southern Germany. In the North, the non-nudists are tolerant to the point of indifference. They take the practice for granted, and *Lichtfreunde* do not suffer in standing or respectability.

In the conservative Catholic South, however, particularly in Bavaria and the southern Rhineland, the feeling is bitter. *Nacktkultur* still has to battle hostile opinion and defend itself against powerful offensives. Nudists caught "practising" on unauthorized territory are not treated with the same leniency as in the North; they can expect severer penalties than a three-mark fine.

Adolf Koch calls his school in Ludwigshafen "an outpost in Bavaria, the Land of the Blackest Reaction." As a matter of fact, there are quantities of "outposts" of *Nacktkultur,* though perhaps not socialist ones. The South has many parks for free physical culture, and Munich in particular is a centre for them. The difference between the North and South is not so much in the number of nudists in the two sections as in the greater prejudice in the South that places more obstacles in their path.

Although the movement is more extensive in Germany than elsewhere, it long ago crossed the boundaries of that country. As early as 1905 there were 103 *Nacktkultur* societies federated in Germany, Austria and Switzerland. A number of the German associations have affiliated clubs in Vienna, such as the *Bund der Lichtfreunde* and the *Gruppe Freie Menschen.* There is also an Austrian league, *Gesunde Menschen,* with centres in Vienna and Linz.

In Hungary, the movement is getting started. There is a park near Budapest, and a semi-nudist centre, on the order of the naturist colony on the Seine, is to be founded.

In Switzerland, the movement has taken on considerable impetus. The *Schweizerische Lichtbund,* with headquarters in Berne, has active groups not only in that city but in Zurich. This society publishes a magazine, *Die neue Zeit,* with unusually fine illustrations, showing hardy mountaineers clambering over Alpine rocks or skiing in the snow fields, innocent of even a loin cloth, and apparently as happy and comfortable as they would be on a tropical isle.

German federations also have affiliated clubs in the chief Swiss cities, such as the *Bund für Freie Lebensgestaltung,* which has a branch in Bâle. The movement's activities, however, are not confined to German Switzerland. At Agnuzzo near Lugano, almost in Italy, is a *Freilichtheim,* with a park and bathing beaches for nudists.

In the North, *Nacktkultur* has spread into the Low Lands. Holland has its movement, and many of the German periodicals carry pictures taken in Dutch nudist camps. In

Belgium likewise it is progressing, though it is there as much an offshoot of the French as of the German movement, for some of the Belgian centres are affiliated with the *Amis de Vivre* of Paris.

We have already discussed the scope of the movement as we found it in France. But the *Amis de Vivre* is growing so rapidly that six weeks after we left there they had added four new branches. The Nice and Toulon centres are now organized and looking for parks in which to meet. Bordeaux announces that it has an enclosed and wooded estate with a villa and camping facilities. Lyons has found an island on a river, with limpid lakes for bathing, woods and large meadows; the members are building a football field and pavilion there. And the Paris group has so flourished that it now has accommodations at its château in Normandy for guests who wish to spend the night, and meals are served to Sunday visitors.

The *Amis de Vivre* are now attempting to organize a group among the students in Paris. We trust that the undertaking will not have the disastrous consequences that would probably follow such a project in a large co-educational university in the United States. Imagine the swift and ruthless action of the Deans of Men and Women who discovered a secret nudist society of undergraduates! The University of Paris, however, is not concerned with the private lives of its students. A student nudist club would probably be unmolested there so long as it did not hold unclad gatherings in the buildings of the Faculties.

More significant still than the progress made by the new centres of *Vivre* is the attention which the practice and theory of nudism are receiving in the general French press. There is no doubt that it is one of the topics of the day.

The popular naturist colony at Villennes has given rise to much of the discussion, for the sketchy costumes of the *Naturistes* at once bring up the question of total versus semi-nudity. The Paris papers have been unable to ignore the thriving island and the doctrines on which it is founded. Articles have appeared recently in the *Journal, Paris-Soir, Paris-Midi, L'Intransigeant,* the Paris edition of the *New York Herald, Comœdia,* and *Gringoire,* among others. Many reporters have visited Villennes, and it is remarkable that a large number of them have found the "music hall" costumes ridiculous and more suggestive than no costume at all.

Two news-reel films, one for the Fox Company, have also been made of the naturists at Villennes.

Some of the journals have published symposiums of the opinions of well-known men and women on nudism. Argument rages pro and con. Typical of many favorable replies is Paul Morand's statement that nudity in the open air is indispensable physically, and that morally it is "the best means of abolishing sexual shame, the troubles of adolescence, perversions, and unhealthy excitations."

The German movement too has been receiving a great deal of attention in France. Three books, the reports of journalists who visited some of the *Freikörperkultur* centres beyond the Rhine, have been published in the last year and a half, and have had enormous sales. One of them, *Au Pays des Hommes Nus,* by L. C. Royer, first appeared serially in *Gringoire,* a popular weekly. All of these books are sympathetic toward the movement, and Roger Salardenne's *Un Mois chez les Nudistes* is an especially sound and comprehensive treatment of the subject. Also a novel on nudism—but French, not German nudism—has appeared, *La Chair au Soleil* by Renée Dunan. The French public, if not converted to the new way of life, at least has heard something about it.

Even England, the European stronghold of Puritanism, is being invaded. Naturally English nudists find many of the same obstacles as they would in America, and they have not much of an organized movement as yet. There is, however, Mr. Faithful's Priory Gate School in Norfolk, a coeducational school where small children and adolescents are all nude.

Parmelee's *Nudity in Modern Life*, or *The New Gymnosophy*, with a preface by Havelock Ellis, has just appeared. A translation of Hans Surén's *Die Mensch und die Sonne* was brought out in England with the original illustrations—clear and unmistakable photographs of undressed men and women. It is noteworthy that Dean Inge of St. Paul's, who was consulted about the morality of publishing it, recommended that it be issued *with the pictures*. In an article "Costume and Custom," printed in the *Evening Standard* October 19, 1927, he not only defended the morality of the book but made pertinent remarks on conventional standards of modesty.

There is also a Gymnosophical Society, recently founded. It does not, or cannot, openly put the nudist doctrines into practise, but the members study such questions as the hygiene of sun- and airbathing, the physiological and educational aspects of nudity, and German *Nacktkultur* and its place in modern life.

In addition to the countries with an organized nudist movement, there are a number with nudist practices so integrated into the customs of the populace that a "movement" is not necessary. Scandinavia is an example. It is well known that in Sweden and Norway men and women bathe together without swimming suits.

An incident that occurred in the French Alps a few years ago illustrated how taken-for-granted such practices are to the Scandinavians.

A group of American, English and French young people, chaperoned by two American matrons, went for a picnic and swimming party on a lonely little mountain lake. One of the guests, a Norwegian army lieutenant, arrived late; the others had finished their swim. He too wanted to bathe, but remarked that he had no suit. The other men offered to lend him one, and when none was found to fit, he said that it did not matter. The others assumed that he had given up the idea of a swim, when a few minutes later he strolled down to the lake, through the midst of the party. To the amazement of the younger people and the horror of the American mothers, he was clad in nothing but his skin. When some of the young men explained to him the consternation he had occasioned, he was extremely surprized and sincerely grieved that he had shocked anyone.

In Finland too, the only European country "moral" enough to have alcoholic prohibition, naked bathing is common. So it is in Russia, and the practice is not one of the radical innovations of the Soviet. Under the Czars, the aristocracy bathed without suits at the fashionable beaches on the Black Sea.

There may be reasons why *Nacktkultur* as a movement should have originated and made its greatest progress in Germany, but none why it should remain confined to that country. Its exportation abroad has already started, and from all indications it is likely to increase in the future.

For one thing, there is no small number of foreigners visiting and even spending extended vacations in the German nudist centres. At Klingberg many nations have been represented. We were not the first Americans—there were two the summer before. The first inscription in Herr Zimmermann's guest book is written in French, and there are testimonials in Danish, Swedish, Dutch, English (even Scotch dialect), Italian and Chinese. Still more nationalities are represented than this would indicate, for there were Austrians and Swiss who wrote in German, and Belgians and even a Luxembourgeois who wrote in French. When we left, Herr Zimmermann had reservations made for another American couple, an Englishman, an Australian, two Parisians, a Frenchman from Morocco, a Belgian, a Hollander and a Hungarian.

It is probable that some of these converts will help spread the new gospel in their own lands. If nothing else, they certainly disprove the accusation that *Nacktkultur* is adapted only to Teutons. Here is the reaction of an Italian as registered in Herr Zimmermann's guest book:

> "To an Italian, proud of his Roman tradition, nudism appears as an artistic return to the pagan glorification

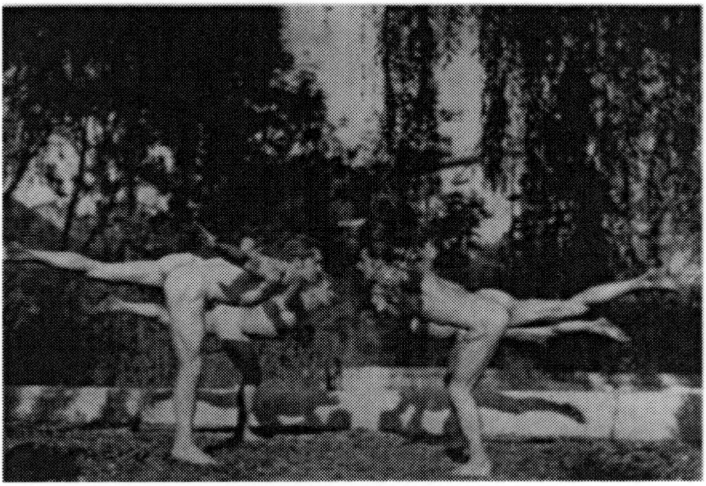

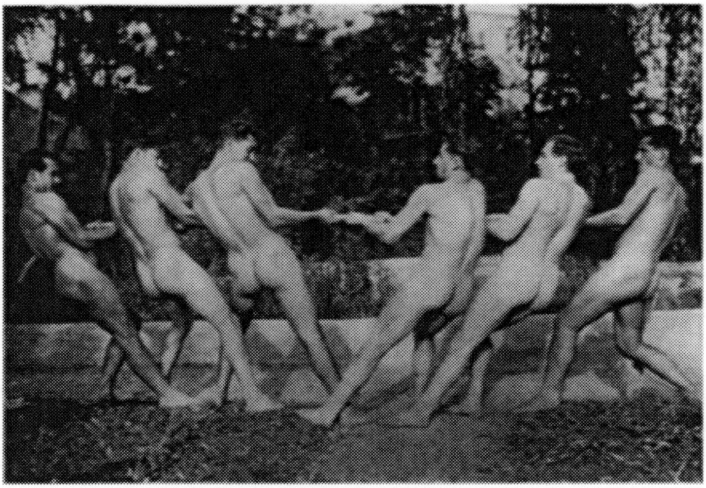

of life for the sake of the beauty of the body and the mind."

Eventually, too, books on the subject will reach the countries that still know little of *Nacktkultur,* just as Surén's book has already reached England. It is possible that the propaganda and missionaries of the cause will be received with indifference, but more likely that there will be persecutions and conversions.

At any rate, nudism has already become sufficiently international for an International Congress. One was held June 8 and 9, 1930, in Frankfurt-am-Main. Delegates attended from eight nations: Austria, England, France, Germany, Holland, Hungary, Italy and Switzerland, with France having by far the largest number of representatives among the foreign countries. Between three and four hundred people altogether were present. Reports were made on the movement in the various countries represented, and such topics discussed as nudity and health, hygiene in general, nudity and morality, and the education of children.

The sessions were held in the open air at one of the nudist parks near Frankfurt, and some of the delegates camped there, while a restaurant set up on the grounds served meals. Recreation was not lacking; there were gymnastic demonstrations and games. Needless to say, the delegates were in uniform—their own bare skins.

It was decided to hold the International Congress annually, at the time of the Whitsuntide holidays, each year in a different country. The 1931 assembly is to meet in France.

XV

THE PHILOSOPHY OF NUDISM

Nudity and Health

THE POINT OF DEPARTURE FOR THE NUDIST MOVEMENT is the importance of sun and air to the health. Nakedness, as we shall see, is advocated for other than physical reasons, but it is characteristic of our scientific age that the nudist philosophy—for it may well be called a philosophy if the word is taken to mean an ordered system and rule of life—has its origin in the discoveries of science.

Adolf Koch gives three sources for the German *Freikörperkultur* movement: the *Schönheitsbewegung* (Beauty Movement) about 1900; the *Jugendbewegung* (Youth Movement), which has been seeking new forms of life; and the *Naturheilbewegung* (Natural Healing Movement), which he defines as tending toward cure without drugs, life in accordance with natural laws, and health through air, water and sunlight. Of these three, it is the last of course that is the most important.

Nacktkultur as only an outgrowth of a Beauty Movement

attempting to improve the body æsthetically, and as a development of a Youth Movement looking for freedom and a better civilization than that of the older generation, would never have reached the tremendous proportions it has in Germany today. It would not, in such a brief time, have penetrated all classes of society and been adopted by the practical materialists as well as the æsthetes, the old as well as the young, and the conservatives as well as the liberals. The strength of *Nacktkultur* is its foundation in medical science.

The use of sun and air in modern therapy is almost too familiar to require emphasis. Violet rays are as characteristic of medicine today as vitamins. Although knowledge of the properties of ultra-violet rays and scientific analysis of the sun's spectrum are comparatively recent, the curative qualities of the sun were known in antiquity. "It seems probable," says Dr. R. C. MacFie, "that ancient Babylonians, Assyrians and Greeks used sunbaths."

It is certain that Hippocrates prescribed sunbaths. "He shall wash himself a very little with warm water, but after having washed, he shall warm himself in the sun," and "very little warm water but exposure to the sun"—these are prescriptions of the Father of Medicine.

The Father of History, Herodotus, has also left testimony on Greek heliotherapy. "Exposure to the sun," he says, "is eminently necessary for people who need to recuperate and take on flesh. . . . As far as possible, one should arrange in winter, spring and autumn for the sun to strike the patients directly; but in summer, this method should be rejected for weak people on account of the excessive heat.

It is the back especially which should be exposed to the sun and fire, for the nerves that obey the will are principally to be found in that region, and if these nerves are in a state of gentle warmth, the whole body is rendered healthy."

The Roman baths, and even private houses, had a special room reserved for sunbaths, a solarium. Pliny the Younger relates that the elder Pliny, who said in his *Natural History* that "The sun is the best of the remedies which one can apply to oneself," was accustomed after his noon meal to lie in the sun while someone read to him. Celsus recommended sunbathing for all delicate people, among whom he numbered "a great part of the inhabitants of cities and almost all men of letters."

In Mediæval medicine—that strange jumble of sorcery, astrology and smatterings of real science preserved by the Arabs—heliotherapy had small place. Nevertheless, one of the Arab physicians, Rhazès, treated smallpox with red light in the ninth century, and a few centuries later sunlight was used in Italy to purify clothes infected by the plague. St. Thomas Aquinas, in the thirteenth century, found that solar radiations were "the necessary condition of plant and animal life."

It was not until the modern era that the use of light and air in healing was established on a scientific basis. Toward the end of the eighteenth century, Faure, La Peyre and Le Comte in France treated ulcers with the sun's rays. At this period, says MacFie, "many books and treatises dealing with the therapeutic value of sunlight were published."

As for airbaths, we find their benefits were discovered

about the same time by no less a discoverer than Benjamin Franklin. July 28, 1760, he wrote to M. Dubourg from London:

> "I greatly approve the epithet which you give, in your letter of the 8th of June, to the new method of treating small-pox, which you call the *tonic* or bracing method; I will take occasion from it to mention a practice to which I have accustomed myself. You know the cold bath has long been in vogue here as a tonic; but the shock of the cold water has always appeared to me, generally speaking, as too violent, and I have found it much more agreeable to my constitution to bathe in another element, I mean cold air. With this view I rise almost every morning, and sit in my chamber without any clothes whatever, half an hour or an hour, according to the season, either reading or writing. This practice is not in the least painful, but, on the contrary, agreeable; and if I return to bed afterwards, before I dress myself, as sometimes happens, I make a supplement to my night's rest of one or two hours of the most pleasing sleep that can be imagined. I find no ill consequences whatever resulting from it, and that at least it does not injure my health, if it does not in fact contribute much to its preservation. I shall therefore call it for the future a *bracing* or *tonic* bath."

So Franklin, a forerunner on so many subjects, seems to have been the first American apostle of nudism. A German nudist, writing in *Soma,* bestows that honour upon a later American celebrity, entitling his article, "Henry D. Thoreau, *der erste Apostel der Freiluft- und Nacktkultur,"* but he was no doubt unaware of Franklin's advocacy of airbathing.

It was in the nineteenth and twentieth centuries, however, that heliotherapy, or phototherapy—a more accurate term since it includes treatment both by artificial light and by the rays of the sun—really came into its own. In 1815, Cauvin in France advocated the sun cure for "all asthenic maladies." The highlights in the history of modern phototherapy, according to MacFie in his *Sunlight and Health,* are briefly these:

Rosenbaum (1835) advised sunbaths for rickets and scrofula. Arnold Rikli (1855) started an institution for sunbaths at Vildes in the Oberkrain. Downes and Blunt (1876) demonstrated that violet light was fatal to bacteria. Finsen used violet light to kill the tubercle bacilli in cases of lupus. Dr. O. Bernhard in St. Moritz (1902) used light successfully in surgical diseases. Rollier at Leysin, Switzerland, and Sir Henry Gauvain in England treated surgical tuberculosis by the same means and their results attracted great attention. Huldschinsky (1919) showed that rickets could be cured by sunlight and even more rapidly by artificial ultraviolet rays.

But sun- and airbaths have not remained cures, to be used only as remedies for specific diseases. Many people believe, and experience seems to bear them out, that these are beneficial for the healthy and normal; the body is strengthened and disease warded off by the increased metabolism resulting from airbathing, and sunbaths effect a reduction of blood-pressure, relief from congestion, increase in the power of the blood to kill disease germs, and retention of phosphorous and calcium.

If we should not wait until children have rickets before supplying their diet with vitamin D, or until we have scurvy before eating food containing vitamin C, why should we wait until we have surgical tuberculosis before letting sun and air reach our bodies? It is the extension of sun- and airbathing beyond the province of treatment for the ill to that of preventive hygiene that is significant in the nudist movement.

Aside from all chemical and physical action of violet rays on the body, a marked psychological effect has been noted. This is highly important in view of the close connexion—stressed in modern medicine—between mental and physical conditions. Exposure to light is immensely stimulating to the mentally depressed, to the neurotic and the anæmic, to all those suffering from melancholy, worry, lassitude and insomnia. We can personally testify from our experience in Germany that troublesome thoughts melt away in a sunbath and are replaced by peace of mind and a sense of contentment and well-being.

The Encyclopædia Britannica, which, as John Langdon-Davies says in his *Future of Nakedness*, "would hardly exaggerate upon such a matter," notes this property of sunbathing:

> "While properly applied insolation exercises a tonic effect on the body, it has been demonstrated that it is equally stimulating to the mind. The exposed subject is notably more cheerful and exhilarated, and evidence

> has been adduced to show that mental responses are brisker and mental activities more pronounced. . . . Sunlight treatment has its greatest therapeutic value in increasing and maintaining bodily tone and energy —its stimulating effect is seen in increasing fecundity. . . . The range of its usefulness is being rapidly extended, in the main, as an aid to cure rather than as a specific treatment."

The question immediately arises, why sunbaths in complete nudity? Cannot enough benefit be derived from the actinic action of the sun's rays without exposing every inch of skin? It has been demonstrated, however, that the ultra-violets do not penetrate even the lightest and sheerest materials. Science has also demonstrated the importance to the body of the sex glands, the very ones that are cut off from violet rays by the minimum costume demanded by modesty.

A French physician, Dr. Fougerat de David de Lastours, has made extensive experiments in exposing patients—men, women and children—to the sun for fifteen days entirely naked and for fifteen days with drawers of fine white linen. The atmospheric conditions in all cases were the same. His records reveal a greater rise in the weight curve and improved morale corresponding with the periods of complete nudity. As a further check of the action of ultra-violet rays on the ductless glands, he gave sunbaths to patients for fifteen days with only the neck covered by a thin cloth, and for fifteen days entirely naked. The records showed greater improvement during the time that the thyroid was uncovered.

Dr. Lastours is convinced that these experiments indicate

the reason for what other physicians have frequently observed, namely, that complete heliotherapy is more successful than local heliotherapy, even in treating a localized disease. Many authorities consider the pigmentation of the entire body an important factor in curing or warding off illness. Patients who tan thoroughly and rapidly show the greatest improvement.

It is difficult in the case of sunbaths to determine just what part is played by violet rays and what part by the air on the naked body—Franklin's "bracing or tonic bath." A sunbath is necessarily also an airbath. Dr. Leonard Hill and Sir Henry Gauvain, English authorities, believe that the improvement in the health from sunbathing is due largely to increased metabolism from exposure to the air; and Halstead, after experience at the Johns Hopkins Hospital and in the Adirondacks, was inclined to the same opinion.

At any rate, it is certain that exposure to the open air does increase metabolism. MacFie gives a table by Lefèvre that shows greatly increased metabolism in a healthy man naked in the open air over that in the same man clothed, with the same temperatures and velocity of air. The table also shows that the higher the velocity of air, the greater the metabolism.

Clothing creates an artificial atmosphere for the body—warm, humid and stale. The skin plays an important part in regulating body temperature, a function clothing disturbs as it retains the heat and prevents the evaporation of perspiration. In hot weather clothing causes prickly heat, from the soaking of the skin in perspiration that is not evaporated normally. As MacFie says, "Men live in a subtropical, damp climate, under a borrowed skin, and when they shed their skin and lie unclothed in the sun—especially in the Alpine sun—they completely alter the climatic conditions in which they have been living. The air instead of being damp and hot, is dry and cold; the air instead of being stagnant, is in movement."

The ancient Greeks, without knowing anything about metabolism or violet rays, were well aware of the superiority of exercise nude over exercise in clothes. It is common knowledge that their sport costume was none at all, and that the word "gymnastic" comes from *gymnos*, "naked." Hippocrates wrote, "Running in clothes has the same property, but it heats too much, renders the body too humid, and gives less colour, because the body is not cleansed by the air that strikes it but exercises while remaining in the same air."

This opinion of a physician who lived more than two thousand years ago is amazingly close to that just cited from MacFie and the following statement by a contemporary French physician, Dr. Pierre Vachet: "Only nudity of the body permits at the same time ease of movement and complete respiration of the skin, or perspiration—an essential function whose activity clothing suppresses or diminishes, and by which the skin eliminates in the form of sweat a part of the waste that, when accumulated, poisons our organism."

In view of this expert testimony, Greek and contemporary, how unhappy—almost criminal, one might say—the spectacle of girls' gymnastic classes in most American schools and colleges, exercising briskly in ample, pleated bloomers of thick serge, heavy middy blouses, and even stockings!

Bathing suits, too, besides being uncomfortable, are actually harmful to the health. According to Parmelee in *Nudity in Modern Life,* some 300,000 gram calories of heat are required to evaporate the water absorbed by the ordinary scanty modern suit. Most of these calories are drawn from the skin, greatly reducing the warmth and vitality of the body. Hence bathers who dry off in their suits are frequently chilled. At times serious diseases may result, particularly in the region of the loins where the organs are near the surface and where the suit is longest in drying. Such diseases are colic and catarrh of the kidneys and bladder.

If clothing did no more harm than to impede our exercises, shut out violet rays, and prevent the air from circulating on the skin, the case against it would be strong enough. But clothes have been guilty of more; irrational fashions throughout the ages have warped the human figure and, especially in the case of women, have caused veritable deformities.

We all of us know—at least all whose memory goes back to the days of strangled waistlines—of the havoc corsets have wrought among women's vital organs. Round garters, too, have done violence to veins and circulatory systems, and have occasioned, in the case of growing girls, malformations of the legs. A recent offence of undergarments is that committed by the brassières that moulded the "boyish form"; too tightly bound, they have actually injured the muscles of the breast. Tight shoes have deformed countless feet, male as well as female, and high heels have thrown the body out of balance, disturbed the carriage and the proper relationship of the different parts of the body. Men have suffered also from tight collars, garters and belts which, by hindering the circulation of the blood, tax the heart.

The art of the ages shows that the ideal female figure has varied throughout the centuries; the Venus de Milo, Cranach's Venus, Boticelli's Venus, and nineteenth century nymphs were not built alike. A French writer, H. Nadel, demonstrates that not only the ideal but the living women varied in the different periods, and he traces in their changing figures the effect of shifting styles in dress.

Venus de Milo, or her flesh and blood models, wore only light, loose garments; stays did not mould her torso. Hence she has remained a standard of physical perfection through the centuries. Judging from many Mediæval works of art, a round belly characterized the fashionable figure. It is, Nadel points out, as if the tall headdress and veils attached to it had projected the abdomen forward. Cranach's Venus has a slender waist and a protruding abdomen; the corset had appeared. The Renaissance Venus, with her prominent stomach and sway-backed grace, was shaped by whalebone bodices. In the plump legs of Rubens' nymphs, Nadel discovers the furrows of garters, and he rechristens Courbet's Source, "The Ravages of Crinoline."

In tropical climates the harm done by the clothes of western civilization to natives accustomed to nakedness is one of the blackest wrongs charged to our colonizing and missionary activities. It is only too well established that the South Sea Islanders, once a strong and healthy race, have suffered frightful inroads from disease since being dressed. A French

Colonial surgeon, as reported by Dr. Lastours, stated a bitter truth when he said:

> "Colonization is becoming humane. In order to make room, no more poison fire-water, massacres, wholesale or retail slaughters. We have better: preachers, bolts of cotton, then a little pulmonary tuberculosis, and six months later the region is cleaned out—quietly—not a soul left. The colonists can come."

Dr. Lastours goes further. His experience in the tropics has convinced him that clothes in equatorial latitudes are as deleterious to Europeans as to natives. Excessive heat and the much-feared tropical sun are better endured, he believes, by the white man if he takes the hygienic precaution of sun-bathing. He finds there is much more danger from sun stroke clothed than unclothed, and a thorough pigmentation is the best armour against the dreaded noon-day heat. He cites numerous instances of northerners who by means of helio-therapy have overcome the unsettled health, lassitude and mental depression that attacked them in the tropics.

Nudity and the tropics may well seem a logical combination, while one might question nudity in cold climates. It is a common assumption that the primary purpose of clothes is to keep the furless, featherless human warm. Anthropology to be sure does not corroborate this theory, and the naked body, once inured to a cold climate, can stand low temperatures without goose flesh.

In regions of Australia where the winters are bitterly cold, natives wear practically nothing. A classic instance is Charles Darwin's encounter with naked savages in Antarctic Tierra del Fuego. Even Eskimos take airbaths in their icy clime. Nansen said that many of them on the west coast of Greenland have died of consumption because European conventions abolished their airbaths. As evidence that acclimation is the thing, Langdon-Davies cites the American woman who is always shivering in England.

The nudists, however, are not asking us to take off our clothes in our northern winters and go bare in the Arctic. Although some Swiss and German devotees demonstrate that one can ski in comfort without a rag on the body, or that a roll in the snow naked is stimulating to a hardy constitution, even they do not insist that nobody should ever wear clothes. All they urge is that nudity in the open air, whenever conditions permit—most people live in a climate where there is sun and warmth part of the time—is desirable for the sake of the health.

Nudity and Morality

But granted the benefits of nudity to the health, why is nudity in common necessary? Why outrage present conventions and run counter to modesty, the principles, customs, and even the laws of our civilization? Why are not the nudists content to take solitary sunbaths, or—if they must have exercise with unconfined pores—to enjoy sports in groups segregated by sex?

It is obvious that if sun- or airbaths must be taken alone, they become merely an hygienic duty, like bathing in a bathtub. And the chances are that they would be perfunctory, if not neglected altogether, since common decency does not require them in the same way that necessity for cleanliness makes soap and water ablutions imperative. Most of us have little time for indulgence in hygienic duties unless they can be combined with recreation and the time devoted to them be truly a part of our leisure, our social life and distraction.

Nor will nudity in company, but with the sexes segregated, solve the problem. Such a division is unnatural—unless one regards the harems of the Orient as the natural way of life, and the relations of the two sexes as based purely on the reproductive function, with nothing to offer each other but sexual pleasure and offspring.

Even in the Oriental harem, family life is intact; the master of the harem at least is free to enjoy the society of the women of his household and spend his leisure in their company. Segregation of the sexes for nude athletics would separate even the family. With money-making what it is, most people have little enough time to spend with their families or friends. If husbands and wives, brothers and sisters, parents and children—to say nothing of unrelated people who have much to gain from the company and friendship of the opposite sex—have to be separated for unclothed outdoor life, they may well prefer to spend their holidays and week-ends dressed and together. Likely they will swim at the beaches where bathing suits are required rather than disport themselves on nudist strands for men or women only.

Of course if nudity in common were positively harmful, or immoral, or even indecent, the fact that it is more enjoyable than solitary or segregated nudity would be no argument at all, except for those whose philosophy is the veriest Hedonism. But the nudists have what they consider conclusive proof that nudity in common is not harmful or indecent, that on the contrary it is morally profitable. Perhaps the moral gain to our civilization from nakedness would outweigh even the benefits of violet rays.

Nudity in common shocks our modesty. Nakedness in public is not only a legal offence; it violates our ethical principles, for modesty is one of our virtues. But what is the nature and origin of modesty in dress? Why are we ashamed to display our naked bodies or to look upon those of others, except in painting or sculpture? There are, of course, civilized people who are ashamed of even the undraped human figure in art—people who put fig leaves on statues and force painters to trail a drapery about the loins of their nudes—but the majority perhaps can view naked bodies with equanimity in artistic representations though not in flesh and blood.

Throughout most of the Christian era, certain portions of the body have been considered shameful, and a minimum of clothing has been regarded as essential. Nevertheless, standards of modesty in dress have varied from generation to generation during this same Christian era. It was not long ago that female ankles were indecent and ladies' legs unmentionable, but in recent years modest ladies have freely displayed not only ankles but knees. The amount of bare bosom permissible has fluctuated no less than skirt lengths. Though evening dress today is allowed to reveal ladies' backs *in toto,* the same liberty is not given to breasts. Yet there were periods in the seventeenth and eighteenth centuries when the décolleté of virtuous gentlewomen extended to the stomach. During the first French Empire, little more than a century ago, breasts were generously displayed. The common costume of Renaissance gentlemen, the skin-tight hose and decorated braguette, would shock us on our streets today.

Even now, our standards vary with the time of day and place. The conventional beach costume, for instance, is deemed indecent for man or woman on the streets and in offices, shops and classrooms, as would be the customary décolleté of women's evening gowns. But we do have a minimum with which no costume worn in public, whatever the time or occasion, may dispense.

This was not always so, even in civilized epochs. Ancient Greece, of course, is the outstanding example of a high state of civilization that did not blush at nakedness. Herodotus notes as an extraordinary fact that "among certain Barbarian peoples it is an opprobrium to appear naked." It was not only in athletic games that the sight of nudity was common. From Grecian art, as well as literature, we learn that it was frequent even in religious rites. And when the Greeks wore clothing, it was light and loose; their dress was not concealing, though neither did it stress sex characteristics as modern dress has always done. In both Ancient Greece and Rome, there was little difference in the costumes of the two sexes.

Although for the Greeks chastity was not the most important of virtues, and their ethics ranked civic virtue higher, their nakedness is not to be attributed to impurity, or vice versa. The Spartan girl ran naked in the stadium—

it was the Spartans, according to Lecky, who first introduced nudity in athletic games—but she would kill herself if a man touched her. Sexual morality, in fact, cannot be gauged by the amount of clothing; the women of old Turkey certainly wore the maximum covering, yet to us Turkish morals are scandalous.

It is interesting to note that in Hindu philosophy, which is regarded as an elevated system of ethics, the philosophers who reach the final and highest stage of perfection, the *gnanis,* dispense with clothing. The *gnani* must pass through three other stages, each with its appropriate costume, before achieving nudity. Nowadays, according to Parmelee, the *gnanis* wear at least a loin cloth, owing to the prohibition of nudity by British law. Parmelee, in fact, has taken the name "gymnosophy," which he has given to nudism, from the Hindu philosophers whom the Greeks called "gymnosophists" from their custom of going naked.

But the Greeks, of course, were pagans, lofty as we still consider their ethical standards in many respects. It is more surprising to discover instances of Christians appearing naked without opprobrium. The Middle Ages were certainly a devout Christian epoch. Nevertheless, we learn from chivalric romances and epics that one of the hospitable attentions the mistress of a castle or the daughter of the house bestowed on visiting knights was to give them baths, or even to massage them with her own hands. Still more amazing, Petit de Julleville tells us that in the passion plays Christ was often represented "naked as an earthworm." Men and women bathed together at the public baths in German towns up to the time of the Reformation.

The Church Fathers, it is true, inveighed against nakedness, as they did against adornment, and the whole ascetic ideal from which monasticism grew was rooted in the belief that the body was shameful. But the early Church, for the first two or three centuries of its existence, did not stress either the shamefulness of the body or the natural evil in man. In fact, the idea of the shamefulness of the body seems rather to derive from the Old Testament, through St. Paul. Hebrew ethics required that nudity should be covered. Certainly the moral conception of the Protestant Reformation and of Puritanism has a distinct Old Testament colour.

Among Christian sects, the Quakers have ranked high for their ethical standards. Leo Markun, in *Mrs. Grundy,* offers some interesting evidence of the early Quaker attitude toward nudity. In Cromwell's England, he relates, two young Quaker girls "ran naked through the streets of Oxford, denouncing the hypocrisy of the people and calling upon them to abandon their sins. The Quaker chroniclers tell us how modest and virtuous these girls were." This sort of demonstration was not confined to England, but was attempted in Colonial America. "Quaker men and women," according to Markun, "ran naked through the streets of Boston, and forced their way, sometimes in the same clothes of Mother Nature, into the Congregational meeting-houses."

There are even instances of contemporary Christian clergymen, Catholic and Protestant alike, who have endorsed the purity of nakedness. Father Sertillanges, Professor in the Catholic Institute in Paris, says in his *L'Art et la Morale,* "Nudity in itself is chaste as nature; it is holy, being from God, and it does not need to conceal its existence."

Among the Protestants, nakedness has a champion no less prominent than Dean Inge of St. Paul's.

Mention has already been made of the survival today of the custom of both sexes swimming without bathing suits in the Scandinavian countries, Finland and Russia. This custom also existed only fifty years ago among the English on the Isle of Guernesey, according to Juliette Drouet, the mistress of Victor Hugo, who shared his exile. The poet himself adopted the native practice. "English customs are opposed to bathers wearing drawers," wrote Mademoiselle Drouet. "Frenchmen having persisted in wearing this brief costume were jeered and almost stoned by men and women."

Most contemporary civilized people, however, imagine that a sense of decency, along with the necessity of keeping warm, is the origin of clothing. If this were the case, decency must be the less potent motive, since nakedness has persisted in hot climates. Anthropologists studying primitive races have found that the real motive for clothing had nothing to do with decency, and that dress was originally designed rather as ornamentation than to cover shameful parts of the body.

As a result of habitually concealing certain parts, however, a feeling of shame at exposing them grew up quite naturally, since man is always ashamed of anything that is contrary to custom or convention. This explains the fluctuations in the decency of legs and bosoms in our modern eras, as well as the immodesty of the bare face of a Mohammedan woman.

Fraser and Westermarck, and explorers who have discovered primitive races before civilization had modified their customs, present a wealth of material showing the relativity of the sense of shame. The Bororos of South America, for instance, wore headdresses, necklaces, belts and anklets, but left the sexual organs uncovered; and a tribe of the Upper Nile wears only ear-rings. The Fuegian dress, and that of the Massas of Africa, is a cape of animal skins which leaves the front of the body completely bare.

"Modesty depends on the custom of covering or exposing certain parts of the body," writes Forel, formerly Professor of Psychiatry in Zurich, "and people who live in a state of nature are as much ashamed of clothes as we are ashamed of nudity."

"Pious people have tried to make savages modest by clothing them," he says further, "but have only produced the contrary effect. . . . The naturalist, Wallace, found in one tribe a young girl who possessed a dress, but who was quite as much ashamed of clothing herself with it as one of our ladies would be of undressing before strangers. . . . All sentiments of morality and modesty rest on conventionalities. The savage women burst into laughter when the naked companions of Livingstone turned their backs from modesty."

Where the custom of covering the sexual organs exists in primitive civilizations, it frequently arises, according to Fraser, from a taboo, due not to shame but to a belief in magic. The sexual organs are often deified in savage or barbarian cultures, and endowed with supernatural properties that make them taboo; they are covered also to protect them from witchcraft or harmful forces.

Again, the girdles, tassels and fringe of the savage are not merely ornamental; instead of subtly provoking curiosity by concealment, some of the decorations hide nothing, but brazenly emphasize. On this matter, Langdon-Davies is worth quoting.

"Sometimes it was not a fig leaf that was worn," he says, "but a gourd, as, for example, among the pygmies of New Guinea, a very primitive type of humanity. . . . Nobody could suggest that the pygmy Adams were trying to conceal anything.

"It would be possible to fill pages with similar evidence that early man wore the little he thought necessary not because of modesty, which we have no right to attribute to him, but because of a vanity which we can have little doubt he possessed. The too sufficient bamboo of the pygmy and the plainly insufficient tassel of the Australian cannot by any manner of juggling or optimism about human nature be explained as a desire to avoid offending the innate delicacy of the female of the species. To our way of thinking the men would be better without them, for their presence on an otherwise naked body must produce the same effect as one word of italics upon a page of ordinary type."

Westermarck mentions many savage ornaments that serve to attract attention to sexual characteristics, and concludes that where nudity is commonplace, the scantiest clothing is a powerful aphrodisiac. Numerous tribes resort to clothing only for erotic dances; such is the case with the feather aprons of Australian women and those worn by some of the African tribes for corroborree rites. The Mincopies of the Andaman Islands, in British India, go naked except when they don, as an apron, a large leaf for their sexual dances.

The men of Pongo in Northern Nigeria, Langdon-Davies points out, wear clothes but refuse to permit their women to do so, lest this embellishment should lead the men of foreign villages to desire them, and the first gown introduced among the Waja was worn to shreds by young men in quest of wives.

Anatole France in *Penguin Island* satirizes delightfully the role of dress in sexual attraction; when the first young Penguin woman is clothed, she is transformed from an ordinary creature, ignored by the Penguin men, into a lovely mystery, followed by a cortège of intrigued males.

The dress of the Greeks, who were accustomed to nudity, was practically the same for both sexes, as was the case with the Japanese, who were used to nudity in common from the practice of men and women bathing together. While we are shocked by nakedness, the Japanese were shocked by the costume of Western women with its exaggerations of sexual characteristics.

Modern dress like that of the savage stresses the difference between the sexes and serves as a means of attraction in the case of women—for it is the women who must attract in modern civilization. Feminine styles have repeatedly emphasized and exaggerated a woman's secondary sexual characteristics. Manifestations of this tendency are the corset, the bustle, the crinoline and the panniers, the prominent bust that required padding and ruffles, low necks and, after legs became alluring through long concealment, the split and then the short skirt. Now that legs have become so commonplace as to lose their allurement, skirts are coming down again, and once more fashions are accentuating waist-lines, hips and the feminine curves that the dissimulation of the late boyish styles have rendered mysteriously enticing.

"In sexual matters," as Forel has said, "it is always novelty that attracts." So styles change, disclosing now this and now that part of the forbidden fruit, which tempts because we are not accustomed to seeing it in its entirety.

All this evidence seems to indicate that our modesty and concealment of the body have little to do with purity. The concealment, in fact, arouses curiosity and endows nudity with an importance and attraction it does not have in itself, and which is wanting when it is an habitual sight. There is no denying that nudity in our modern civilization has an erotic effect which makes it valuable in pornography and on the music hall stage. The naked body has become almost purely a sexual symbol, owing to the habit of keeping it covered. But even pornography has discovered that partial nakedness is more suggestive than nakedness unadorned, and appreciates the effect of the italics, as Langdon-Davies has it, on a page of ordinary type.

There are people who would regret the disappearance of dress, not only because of their æsthetic appreciation for its possible beauty of colour and line, but for fear that the loss of its erotic stimulation would remove one of the valuable and legitimate pleasures of life. The answer to them is that the nudists do not seek to abolish dress completely, for all occasions. The practice of nudity does not take anything essential from sex feeling; it will not result in an asexual race. It will lead merely to a healthier and more rational attitude on the subject and do away with morbid sexual preoccupations and a shame that is often harmful.

The dangers of the prudery that stimulates curiosity, at times to the point of sexual obsessions and perversions, have been pointed out by Forel. "The sexual sentiment of modesty," he says, "very often becomes unhealthy and is then easily combined with pathological sexual conditions. Prudery is, so to speak, sexual modesty codified and dogmatized. It is indeterminate, because the object of modesty is purely conventional, and man has no valid reason to regard any part of his body as shameful."

For the perils of prudishness, the Swiss psychiatrist has a remedy. "Prudery can be created or cured," he states, "by education in childhood. It may be created by isolation, by covering all parts of the body, and especially by making children regard nudity as shameful. On the other hand, it may be cured by mixed bathing, by accustoming the child to consider the human body, in all its parts and functions, as something natural of which one need not be ashamed, lastly by giving instruction on the relations of the sexes, in due time and in a serious manner."

With these suggestions, nudists would heartily concur, for in the educational value of nudity and its psychological importance lies, they believe, one of the best arguments in its favour and the chief justification for nudity in common, without distinction of age or sex. As Parmelee points out, "To call special attention to the organs of sex by means of the taboo upon nudity is deliberately to incite sexual precocity in the child."

Dr. Pierre Vachet, the French psychiatrist, believes thoroughly in the beneficial effects of nudity and recommends it as a method of education. "The practice of nudism," he says, "would no doubt be the best means of rendering simple and easy the sexual education of the young, while keeping them from the curiosities, the fevers of the imagination, and the incertitude before the sustained mystery that are at the origin of all perversion."

The practice of nudity would also preclude the worry lest they are not developing properly that some children, ignorant of what is normal, experience in adolescence. Ashamed of speaking of these fears, they sometimes suffer veritable torture that may warp their later life. This is particularly true of girls, as boys have more opportunity to see members of their own sex nude.

That nudity, when it is familiar, does not arouse erotic emotions is well known to artists who work from living models and doctors who examine women. Nor does it take them long to acquire this cool indifference to the spectacle of the other sex without clothes. Practical experience, the experience of all, including the writers, who have taken part in nudist gatherings or visited their centres, is the best evidence of the psychological effect of nudity in common.

The visitors to such groups, even those going in the most sceptical frame of mind, have testified to the morality of the nudists as well as to the quickness with which one grows accustomed to the sight of nakedness. "The sexual question seems to play no role," remarked the journalist who reported the International Congress of Nudism in *Comœdia* (Paris), June 17, 1930.

The unclothed body rapidly becomes commonplace,

neither shameful nor erotically stimulating. The prudery and curiosity, fostered by the training of a lifetime, vanish in a few hours. The modest are astonished at not being shocked, and those seeking a pornographic feast are disappointed. In fact, if nudism should become universal, pornography would suffer tremendously.

As Nadel has said, the sexual idea evoked by nakedness is a "simple association of images. When nudity will be frequently encountered, when men work naked, play naked, live naked, it will not evoke one act more than another. The body will cease to be a sexual fetich and will once more take on its real value."

Even the Doctors Durville, who insist that France is not ready for nudism as is Germany, recognize the calming effect sexually of total nudity in common. They believe, however, that for the Germans, in spite of the fact that they are as highly sexed as the French, nudity and sexuality are two different things, while for the French they are but one, and these doctors urge the necessity of "educating France in nakedness." They themselves have cured patients of sexual obsessions by means of the practice of nudity, and they look forward to a day when "the new man reaccustomed to the atmospheric elements will see his sexuality police itself."

This is by no means a discovery of the contemporary nudists. The artist Gauguin noted it in connexion with the South Sea Islanders. In his *Noa Noa* he said, "Their continual state of nakedness has kept their minds free from the dangerous preoccupation with the 'mystery' and from the excessive stress which among civilized people is laid upon the 'happy accident' and the clandestine and sadistic colours of love. It has given their manners a natural innocence, a perfect purity."

Senancour, the author of *Obermann,* in a book on love published in 1806, devoted a chapter to nudity. According to Parmelee, he believed that nudity would diminish passion but would enrich the sentiment of love in other respects.

Nudity and Beauty

No doubt vanity is, after all, a greater obstacle to the nudist movement than modesty or shame. In view of the decorative origin of dress, and the important role it still plays in attraction, it is not to be wondered at if women particularly should be unwilling to abandon such a potent method of enhancing their charms. Most men and women are painfully aware of their physical shortcomings and appreciate the advantages of what Nietzsche called the "masquerade" of clothing. Many, too, who have no reason to be ashamed of their own bodily endowments, shuddering at the thought of the ugliness that would be revealed if all humanity were naked, oppose nudity on æsthetic grounds.

The perfect body, of course, is not ugly, or artists would never have set up the well-formed human figure as an ideal of beauty, and time and time again have devoted themselves to its representation. Anyone who finds the masterpieces of Greek sculpture ugly is in a pathological condition. It is true unfortunately that few of our contemporaries even approach the classical standards of physical perfection. There are people, the extremely misshapen—after all com-

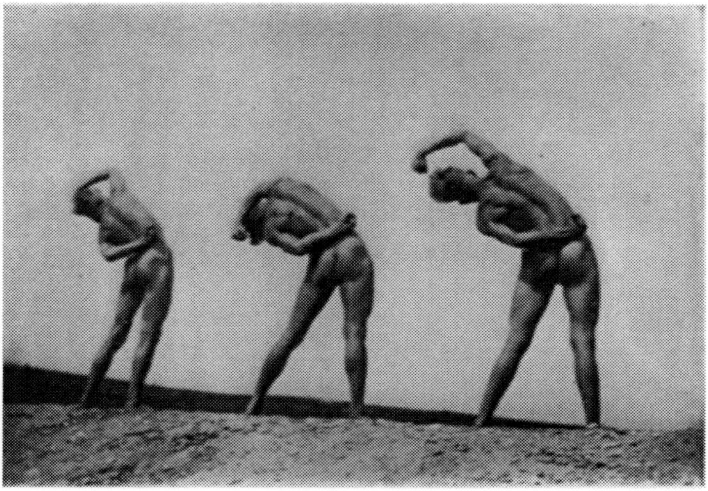

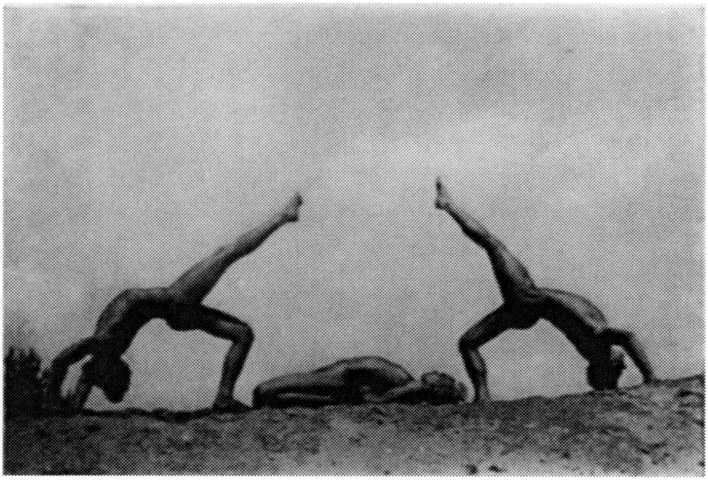

paratively few—who are better to look at with some kind of covering, no matter how inartistic or ridiculous that covering may be. Others undoubtedly gain by being undressed, those who have healthy, symmetrical bodies but plain, or downright homely, faces, or those who dress in such a way as to obscure their physical attractions.

For it cannot be assumed that clothes are necessarily attractive, any more than are bodies. Some styles are absurd or hideous—as we can usually appreciate when they have ceased to be in style—and even when the fashions themselves are æsthetically pleasing, there are always plenty of people, probably the majority, who are too careless, or too lacking in taste, or too poor, to dress in a becoming manner. We all know what a world of difference there is in the appearance of the elegant lady endowed with taste and wealth and that of the ignorant working girl with cheap tastes and no wealth, though both have the same fashions and the same desire to be attractive.

Most people are neither beautiful nor ugly without clothes; they are mediocre, just as are the majority when dressed. They may not arouse admiration, but they are an inoffensive spectacle. Maurice Parmelee, who has had much experience in nudist centres, thinks that the practice of nudity discloses more beauty than ugliness. A completely beautiful or harmonious body is rare, but the greater number have some good features.

Also, it is more than likely that the feeling many have of the ugliness of the naked form would be considerably modified once all idea of shame or evil associated with the body had been dispelled. Even people who consider themselves emancipated, and who recognize rationally that there is nothing shameful in nakedness, cannot avoid having their emotional reactions coloured unconsciously by the conventions according to which they were reared. The practice of nudity in common would rid them of this feeling as no amount of theory or reasoning could.

Dr. Gaston Durville has still another explanation for the painlessness of the spectacle of our naked fellow men. In describing an extremely fat woman he saw, both dressed and undressed, at the International Congress in Frankfurt, he said: "Naked, she is no more ridiculous, no uglier; indeed she is even less so. I have several times observed similar instances. Perhaps this optimistic impression is due to the fact that when one is showing one's own imperfections, one becomes more indulgent toward those of others. Total nudity is a school of humility."

Furthermore, the very practice of nudity increases the beauty of the body. Nor is it necessary to wait long for the first improvement. Although the body on being released from its wrappings may look sickly, anæmic and pale, merely a brief exposure to the sun will give the skin a beauty exceeding that of the most delicate, sheltered, lily-white complexion. Pigmentation, quite aside from its therapeutic value, is pleasing to the eye. The warm tints of brown and tan give a healthy impression and clothe the body, as it were, in a natural and becoming dress. One of the things that struck us in the nudist centres was the greater attractiveness and harmony of the tanned skins; beside them, the white bodies, newly emerged from their swaddlings, were unnatural and almost indecent. We were conscious that they were "undressed," while we did not think of clothes in connexion with the dark bodies.

It is a common experience on returning to the city from a country place or resort where everybody was more or less bronzed to notice the pale tint of the urban dwellers and to feel that they are all unhealthy. We realize, too, what a difference a tanned face can make in the appearance. You return from a few days in the country, and although you may not have been there long enough for your health to benefit in any way, although you may be just as thin, just as tired and nervous as before, nevertheless, if your complexion is browned, your friends will exclaim, "How well you are looking!" They will even insist that you have gained weight. Michelet realized this years ago and wrote of the young woman of his day, "Everything would be gained if her white skin were turned to the living brown tones."

With exposure to the sun and air, the skin also becomes smoother and more silky, and many little blemishes vanish. There is no doubt that it is toughened so as to withstand irritations that would roughen or break a delicate skin. Men whose faces are tanned on a vacation, provided of course they are not burned, have discovered this in shaving.

Dr. Fougerat de Lastours describes the æsthetic benefits of nudity in the open air. "The skin becomes healthy, takes on colour of a warmer patina, the tint of health. The muscles assume fuller or less abrupt contours, the lines are softened, the whole gains in strength and grace, the body develops harmoniously and acquires a beauty that any other method is powerless to give without the aid of exposure to the sun."

The beauty imparted by naked outdoor life is indeed more than skin deep. Sunbathing and exercise in the open air naturally strengthen the body and give it the beauty that can come only from health. Although after maturity there is not much we can do about our bones, we can do a great deal about flesh and our posture and carriage. There is no greater incentive to improvement in these matters than nudity in common. Out of carelessness and inertia, we neglect defects more or less hidden under clothes, but when we must remove the sartorial screen and disclose ourselves to the public, our complacency is shaken.

One nudist society with numerous branches states in its constitution, according to Parmelee, "that members who become excessively corpulent are to be suspended. This measure is in part for æsthetic reasons, but also is a penalty for an unhygienic mode of life."

Hence, in spite of the unloveliness of humanity on first discarding its garments, there is hope for its rapid embellishment. This prospect is particularly bright for the generation following the pioneers in nudity. For if children are brought up according to nudist doctrines from birth, they should be physically stronger and more graceful; clothes will neither warp their figures nor serve as a masquerade for remediable defects.

The improvement of the race in both health and beauty, as well as morality, is a goal toward which the nudists aspire. "What better epitaph could a simple man require," asks Langdon-Davies in his witty speculations on *The Future of Nakedness,* "than some such words as these: 'He helped us to take off our clothes'?" He adds, "And if such an epitaph as this can be honestly earned by him, the writer of this little book at least will be able to die happily."

There is one more objection advanced at times against the nudist theory. Some worry lest nakedness set up standards by which the stupid and beautiful should be preferred to the brilliant with wretched physiques. Since the most perfect physical specimens are often far from being the worthiest or the most intelligent, this concern is comprehensible. But have clothes prevented us from giving beauty, even a factitious beauty derived from artifices in dress, an unfair advantage? In a society of naked men and women artificial beauty at least has no chance.

What the nudists seek, however, is the combination of the two things, the beautiful mind in the beautiful body. A fervent French nudist leader, Charles-Auguste Bontemps, the editor of *Vivre,* expressed what is undoubtedly the opinion of most intelligent nudists when he said that he would always prefer the intelligent physical weakling to the stupid man with the body of a Greek god, even while holding to the ideal of beauty in both body and mind. To dispel the fear that the two are incompatible, one need only remember that the Greek devotion to physical perfection did not impair the mentality of the race.

Nudist Attitudes

In a discussion of nudist theory, a word perhaps on the relation of nudism and naturism would not be amiss, since the two are often confused.

The naturists, advocating a life in accordance with natural laws, consider the practice of nudity a useful hygienic measure, though not the most important. They generally believe that a strictly vegetarian diet and abstention from alcohol, tobacco, and drugs—even the mildest of medicines—are more essential to the health. Hence some of them are willing, as is the case of the *Société Naturiste* in France, to sacrifice total nudity to the requirements of convention.

The nudists may or may not be naturists; many of them in Germany are naturists, but the majority are not. The Durvilles criticize the German nudists for destroying all the beneficial effects of a week-end in a *Nacktkultur* park by a huge meal of sausages and beer on their return. The nudists, as distinct from the naturists, while recommending a sane and temperate life, put their faith primarily in nudity and physical culture. They do not urge a return to nature; they wish man to remain a civilized being, discarding nothing that is an improvement on nature merely because it is artificial. But they want him to profit as fully as possible from the benefits of light and air—his need for them, as a result of urbanism and the rapid tempo of modern life, being imperative.

Nor do they advocate compulsory nudity. They are not prohibitionists of clothes—and wisely, since clothing, with all its decorative value and erotic effect, would certainly be bootlegged at our present stage of civilization. One can imagine the clandestine dens of vice that would spring up, places where the patron could see dressed people, and in the worst ones, even dress himself! "It is the part of wisdom," says one of the most enthusiastic preachers of nudist doctrines, Parmelee, "to utilize clothing whenever it is needed, and not to misuse it when more can be gained from going without."

All the nudists ask is tolerance for their doctrines, respectability for nakedness, and the right to undress without interference and scandal. Their example and education, they believe, will do the rest.

XVI

AMERICA AND NUDITY

DOES THE NUDIST MOVEMENT HAVE A FUTURE IN AMERICA? Is there any likelihood that it will penetrate our boundaries, as it has those of France; or even a remote possibility that it will assume the proportions here it has in Germany? Doubtless many will categorically answer "No."

Yet it is pertinent to ask whether our conventions and customs are endangered by the peril of nakedness, for many people will likely consider it a peril. Certainly the garment industry would look on nudism as a subversive doctrine, to be combated by every means that the textile manufacturers, the clothing makers, and the bathing suit companies—to say nothing of the laundries and dry cleaners—can mobilize. In the United States we always have to reckon with the influence of big business. We can imagine the colossal struggle that might ensue between the clothing interests and the advocates of nudity, marked by all the features, the lobbying, purchase of newspapers and subsidizing of educators, that have characterized the battle of the power trusts with the advocates of government ownership of utilities.

If the nudists should win out—if, as Langdon-Davies asserts, "it will indeed be a short time only before a person who wears more than a loin cloth on Fifth Avenue will be stigmatized as indecent and degenerate,"—we point out for the consolation of industry the opportunities in anti-sunburn oil and sandals, as well as pouches and handbags to replace pockets.

But, quite aside from the possible opposition of business, and in spite of Langdon-Davies' optimism about the future dress of Fifth Avenue, there are serious obstacles to the progress of nudism in America. That state of mind we call Puritanism, or Anglo-Saxon prudery, is undeniably prevalent in this country, and it is certain to be shocked into action by nudism. We have only to read the catalogues of countless denominational colleges of numerous religious sects to realize the horror with which many of our compatriots regard such limited exposure of nakedness as that of short sleeves and low necks, as well as their fear of allowing the young of the two sexes to associate even far less freely than in a nudist centre.

Large numbers of Americans, as everyone knows, are also opposed to nudity in art, particularly outside of art galleries—for the nude exhibits of the Metropolitan and other museums seem to be accepted with calmness. A nude statue on a public square, or a nude painting in a public building, frequently has a sad fate in this country. That the Wisconsin legislators forced Kenyon Cox to superimpose a scrap of floating drapery on an allegorical figure in the mural decorations of the Senate Chamber in the State Capitol is neither surprising nor unique. On the other hand, the protectors of morals do not always prevail: witness the defeat last summer, by the firemen and Chief of Police, of the lady in Winona Lake, Indiana, who attempted to dress in poison ivy a reproduction of the Venus de Milo.

These campaigns against nudity in art are by no means peculiar to America. Statues and paintings have been attacked on moral grounds and even mutilated in European countries, including the nation with the greatest reputation for tolerance of indecency—France. Carpeaux's group, "The Dance," on the Paris Opera, was splattered with ink by a prude, and Houdon's "Diana" was refused by the Salon for too great realism in the indication of sex. In Germany, as recently as last August, the Minister of the Interior of Thuringia forbade the use of nude models in the art school of Weimar, stipulating that all models posing for life classes should wear bathing suits.

This demonstrates that although a Germany made up of Thuringian ministers of the interior would have no *Nacktkultur,* the existence of such an attitude in a country does not preclude authorized nudism within its borders. Since America is not made up exclusively of ladies who drape Venus in poison ivy, but has also heroic firemen who by turning on their hose uproot the ivy, we too might be receptive to nudism in spite of our moral crusaders.

The attitude exemplified by the small denominational colleges of the Southwest is by no means universal; American youth, by and large, associates rather freely with the other sex, and more girls wear short sleeves and low necks when the latter are in style than do not wear them. To the sorrow of many, our Puritan moral fibre has been seriously warped. Taken as a whole, we are probably more shockable than the French, but not more so in regard to nudity than the French bourgeoisie. And we have seen that in spite of their modesty on the subject, nudism is growing in France.

Nevertheless, we do have more blue laws than does the French Republic. It is characteristic that many of our public beaches have more stringent regulations in regard to bathing costumes than those abroad, and still prohibit stockingless legs for women and one-piece bathing suits. Eighteen youths were fined a dollar apiece one day last summer for letting down their bathing suits at Coney Island in order to tan their chests. They did not, said the magistrate, "take the women into consideration." At the same time nine were fined for wearing bathing suits in the streets—a further demonstration of the relativity of modesty in dress.

Countless of our tourists have gasped at the spectacle of fashionable French beaches. They have been distressed to find that they could not rent anything there more modest than a flimsy one-piece garment of cotton, and ladies have discovered that to persist in wearing stockings only attracted the embarrassing scrutiny of the crowd.

In France, and even in Germany, particularly Southern Germany, nudity in public does bring legal chastisement. American police could do no more to prevent indecent exposure than the French police of Grenoble a few years ago. When a group of students, fully clothed, gave a fellow student, also fully clothed, a bath in a fountain, the officers of the law arrested not only the culprits and their victim but all innocent bystanders who were watching the fun, on the grounds that they probably would take off their clothes. The whole crowd, including the bystanders, spent the night in jail.

But more formidable as an obstacle to nudism than the mere existence of laws is the undoubted presence in America of many people who would regard the conduct of nudists as their business, and who would take it upon themselves to report it to the authorities. Whether owing to a greater sense of civic responsibility on the part of our countrymen, or to a greater propensity for "snooping" and meddling, this trait is characteristic of many Americans, and it would greatly hamper the practice of nudity. Langdon-Davies notes this and contrasts it with customary English behaviour.

"It is, indeed, really quite astonishing," he says, "to what lengths the American public will go in their zeal against nakedness, especially if it extends beyond arms and shoulders and legs; and even in California one meets with almost Quixotic examples of this zeal, as, for instance, when quite a number of people hurrying home to their beds two hours after midnight delayed themselves to telephone to the police when they saw two naked forms about to enter the surf."

"Of course it is very creditable to the American sense of citizenship," he continues; "in England, we fear, most of us would either have stopped and watched, or gone home to bed; few would have wasted a small coin and precious minutes, which might be spent asleep, on such a public service."

An outraged Englishman might, though Langdon-Davies does not say so, write a letter about the affair to the *Times* next morning, but neither he nor anyone else would actually expect the *Times* to do anything about it. We, on the contrary, expect somebody to do something, and if the police fail us we rely on our Watch and Ward or Anti-Vice Societies to set the matter right. Such organizations, and likely the Ku Klux Klan—nudism being of foreign origin—might conceivably have a good deal to do about nudists.

The reactions of our friends and other people to whom we have spoken of the nudist movement are perhaps significant of what will be the attitude of many Americans. For, superior as we like to think our associates, they are without doubt typical Americans; in fact, we must admit that they belong to a class in no way exceptional—the large middle class—that is both the stronghold of respectability and the backbone of the nation.

The first reaction, naturally enough, is one of bewilderment and incredulity. People are too stunned to do more than gasp and blink, though some recover from the shock much more rapidly than others. Some never do recover, such as an editor with whom we attempted to discuss the possibility of articles on *Nacktkultur.* Throughout our interview, his face expressed utter terror; apparently he feared that at any moment we might become violent and take off our clothes in his office.

But most people, once we have succeeded in making clear the nature and extent of the movement, are ready to consider it seriously and to discuss it calmly, conceding advantages and raising rational objections. They display considerable diversity of opinion, and it is not always possible to predict what the attitude of various persons will be. A liberal and emancipated young intellectual may be strongly opposed to the idea, while a conventional spinster from a prudish background may accept it enthusiastically. On the whole, however, there is a certain amount of agreement in the viewpoints of these various people. The advantages of nudity to the health are generally granted, though with a difference in the degree of importance assigned to them. And those to whom we have talked have been unanimous in endorsing swimming without bathing suits, at least in privacy.

It is nudity in common, of course, rather than nudity itself, that arouses opposition—generally, but by no means exclusively, on moral grounds. A few people have said at once that nudity is in no way dangerous to morality, that it is purer than semi-undress, but the most frequent question—as is to be expected in view of the connotations of nakedness in our civilization—is about the erotic effect of nudity in common. Does it not lead to all kinds of libertinism? Do not people, at the sight of the unaccustomed nakedness of the opposite sex, become excited? And, if the nudist centres are as moral as we say, is it not due to a temperamental difference in the German people?

Of course, it is only necessary to cite the night life of Berlin to show that the Germans are not essentially less erotic or purer sexually than other peoples.

At the other extreme are those, generally rather liberal and well informed, who immediately concede the purity of nudity, but who fear that it will impair, if not completely destroy, sex attraction. An intelligent spinster whose business career and travels have given her a background of varied experience, a young matron who is a writer, and a university instructor who also is married, are among those raising this question.

Mature and enlightened people such as these deserve consideration, but there is less reason to pause at the objections of a collegiate youth who was alarmed lest the practice of nudity make "petting" impossible. Of course, the younger generation could always put on clothes for "petting parties," but lamentation at a decline in this popular modern sport would not be universal.

The value of the practice of nudity in the education of children is often recognized. A physician—incidentally a child specialist—who displayed no little incredulity as to the moral effect of nudity on adults, declared without hesitation when nudity for children was mentioned: "Certainly, that's the only way to bring up kids!" Those also who fear that the practice of nudity, rather than leading to libertinism, will lessen sex attraction and destroy some of the charm of relations between the sexes, advocate the nudist system for children, agreeing that sex emotions and erotic feelings should not be awakened prematurely.

The æsthetic question is brought up frequently, perhaps as frequently as that of morality. Many who readily approve of nudism on hygienic or moral grounds qualify their endorsement with a "provided that everybody is good looking." Some who find even the average human body a pleasant spectacle declare that they would be revolted at the sight of the excessively corpulent or misshapen. Others insist that everybody is more attractive dressed; that nakedness, while not shameful or indecent, is almost invariably ugly.

This opinion can often be traced to the unconscious influence of early education in the belief that nudity is evil. Such is the case of a young woman whose ideas are constantly at variance with her conventional conduct. Intellectually emancipated, she is still governed by the Puritan conscience a strict upbringing instilled in her. She is willing to advocate nudity, in spite of her æsthetic objections, but it.is unlikely that she will ever practise it.

This inconsistency we have found in numerous others; theoretically they are nudists, but they insist they would never put the theory into practice, either from lack of courage to defy custom, or from vanity—for some frankly admit they would refuse to display their physical mediocrity in public.

Of course, if the practice of nudity became general and more or less acepted in this country, the first reason would no longer exist, and the second would become less common on the discovery by many people that they did not compare too unfavourably with others.

The whole idea is so new to most Americans that few of those with whom we talked were able to formulate any opinion immediately. It was only after considerable discussion that they knew what they actually thought about the matter. There were exceptions, however. One was a young man, a professor in a large university, who at once exclaimed, "Fine! I think that's the way back to the Greek ideal." Another was a young woman teaching in a girls' private school who, as soon as she heard such a movement existed, was "green with envy" because she could not go to Germany and join it. Many spoke of enjoying the free feeling of being unclothed and the sensation of light and air, as well as water, on the naked body, although they might be dubious in regard to nudity in common.

Practically all the objections raised in the course of our conversations were those encountered by the movement in Europe. We have already discussed them in connexion with the philosophy of nudism and given the arguments the nudists oppose to them. In this country, we have heard no criticisms—with the possible exception of that of the young collegian—which can be considered peculiarly American, though to be sure we have not had an opportunity to discuss the matter with any of our Southern Fundamentalists or our provincial Main Streeters.

The American public has not yet had an opportunity to take a stand on nudism, and one cannot say that the movement has even begun here. Some of the German *Lichtfreunde* believe it has, for they have heard of an active nudist group in the United States. But this small group, of about sixty or seventy members, affiliated with one of the large German associations, is made up chiefly of German-Americans, and the very existence of the group is unknown to outsiders. Owing to the extra-legal status of their practice, and the fact that they are men and women of standing in their communities, they cannot jeopardize their positions—business or professional and social—by legal proceedings. Hence they have been unable to do much proselytizing. Nevertheless, while their ultimate success cannot be foretold, it is perhaps a hopeful sign that their group has grown and flourished in the single year that they have been organized.

We have had native precursors, it is true, but not only were they isolated figures who made no attempt to formulate a conscious nudist philosophy, but their influence in this direction can scarcely be deemed important. They are all long dead, and still there is no sign of their gospel flowering into a nudist movement. In addition to Franklin and Thoreau, previously mentioned, the only outstanding figure is that of Whitman, who repeatedly sang of the glory and beauty of the human body and of the purity of nakedness. One of his passages in *Specimen Days in America,* as quoted by Parmelee, expresses well the conviction of contemporary nudists:

> "Sweet, sane, still Nakedness in Nature!—ah if poor, sick, prurient humanity in cities might really know you once more! Is not nakedness then indecent? No, not inherently. It is your thought, your sophistication, your respectability, that is indecent. There come moods when these clothes of ours are not only too irksome to wear, but are themselves indecent. Perhaps indeed he or she to whom the free exhilarating ecstasy of nakedness in Nature has never been eligible (and how many thousands there are!) has not really known what purity is—nor what faith or art or health really is."

Parmelee himself, that present-day apostle whose enthusiasm carries him so far as to construct in his *Nudity in Modern Life* a Utopia based on nudist principles, is an American, formerly Professor of Sociology in the University of Missouri, but his message as yet has reached only the English public.

Nevertheless, there are certain factors in American life that might favour the progress of the movement. The most obvious is the popularity of sunbathing in recent years. During the past few summers, whether seeking health or merely a fashionable "sun tan," countless Americans have been toasting themselves. Many are content with the partial brown coat that can be acquired while wearing a bathing suit, but many others take complete, though solitary, sunbaths whenever they can find the requisite privacy. The complete sunbath devotees are probably moved more by the desire for health than by fashion, for the latter still does not sanction revealing the complexion resulting from total exposure.

The healthful properties of ultra-violet rays are familiar in America. Our physicians prescribe them, and the sufficiently affluent purchase artificial sun lamps. Last summer, the Health Commissioner of Chicago made a plea for nude solariums at the public beaches—to be fenced away from prying eyes, of course, and with the two sexes strictly segregated. Such solariums already exist in Florida, and probably elsewhere in this country.

The vogue for sun-bronzed skin has manifested itself not only in "sun-back" bathing suits for both sexes, but in "sun-back" sport dresses and stockingless legs for women. Though the bare-legged fad is apparently receding, its very appearance proves that, traditional modesty notwithstanding, the mode is capable of baring what generations have covered.

The women's styles that have just vanished around the corner—the loose, knee-length tunics requiring neither corsets nor much of anything else beneath them—gave encouragement, not only to nudists but to other believers in practical and hygienic dress. Rash prophets announced that long skirts, ample folds, and corsets would never return. Fashion fooled them. The new styles are a retrogression, hygienically speaking. But fashion being the turncoat she is, there is no need to fear that brief and scanty dress is gone forever.

Numerous Americans are also aware of the joys of bathing without bathing suits. Many of our modest compatriots, who would never dream of appearing unclothed before members of the other sex, no more hesitate about swimming outdoors minus bathing suits, if the spot is deserted, than about bathing in that state in their own bathrooms. Men have long been accustomed to bathing together nude in such highly respectable places as Y.M.C.A. pools, and to dispense with suits at the "Ole Swimmin' Hole" has always been a prerogative of boyhood. In the summer of 1929, when the police arrested a number of youths for exercising the prerogative on the Hudson in the reaches above New York City, there were editorials in New York papers defending the inalienable right of boys to bathe *au naturel.*

Another growing custom—one that is hard to verify but that several people have assured us their friends confess to adopting—is that of sleeping without nightclothes. There is no doubt that the custom is prevalent during excessive heat waves, a fact that can be corroborated from the vantage point of any building facing a hotel on a hot summer night. It is a question here, however, not of a desperate resort of frenzied heat victims, but of an habitual practice in all temperatures—except possibly during the most excessive cold—for the sake of comfort and hygiene. If the custom becomes at all general, it might prove an entering wedge for nudism.

In addition to these rather obvious nudist "tendencies," there are less conspicuously revelant but more fundamental American characteristics that might dispose us to accept the nudist doctrines. In the first place, as a nation we undeniably assign great importance to hygiene. In fact Europeans, sensitive to American boasting on the subject of bathtubs, sometimes accuse us of judging civilization solely on the basis of hygienic progress and of preferring sanitation to art and intellect. Whether or not we are unduly idolatrous in worshipping the Goddess Hygeia, any health measure backed by sufficient authority is bound to be welcome in this country. If enough prominent doctors endorse nudism, there is no doubt of its adoption by many.

Then too, we pride ourselves on being an athletic nation—perhaps somewhat unjustifiably since, though we supply the world with plenty of champions, our athletic enthusiasm is too often that of the spectator, and our automobiles have deprived many of even the gentle exercise of walking. But in spite of our weakness for professional sports and gasoline engines, our secondary schools and colleges regularly require gymnastics and organized athletics, and outdoor exercise thrives in the classes that have sufficient time and money. Practically all of the younger generation who have had any opportunity in life can swim and play some kind of a game of tennis, and practically all of the older men who can afford it play golf. Nudism, as was pointed out to us in Germany, appeals to lovers of sport.

Although too many Americans enjoy nature only through a haze of dust, whizzing bill-boards, and hot-dog stands, something of our pioneer life survives in the popularity of camping and hunting and fishing trips. No other nation resorts so largely in the summer to huts and tents in the woods, and even automobiles are purveyors to roadside camps as well as wayside inns. To live primitively in the heart of nature is the typical vacation of many Americans. Perhaps the distance from nature in khaki and tweeds to nature in naked skin is not too great to be traversed.

Our modern ideas on the education of children also predispose us to taking the step. As psychologists stress the harm that may be done by suppressed curiosity, many young Americans who never thought of nudity in common for adults are accustoming their children to their own nudity and that of their parents, with the definite purpose of developing a rational attitude toward the body and all its parts and functions.

Perhaps too, if prosperity fails to recover soon from its present sickness, our economic depression, with the resultant need for simple, inexpensive amusements, will favour the spread of the nudist movement as it has in Germany. That, however, belongs in the realm of pure speculation.

Of course prophecy is always dangerous. Moreover, in this case, the very fact that we, the writers, have dared to try such a rash thing as nudism will doubtless afford ample proof, at least to many Americans, that we are so lacking in judgment and a sense of proportion that our views are worthless if not pernicious. Nevertheless, of one thing we feel certain: sooner or later the nudist movement in Europe will come to the attention of the American public.

As to the possibilities of its spreading to this country and becoming eventually greater or less in scope than at present in Germany, we shall prudently reserve judgment. As to whether or not it will ever achieve governmental and legal recognition, it is impossible to say, even though Langdon-Davies does assure us that "We shall get rid of our clothes inevitably, because of the contradictions and conflicts inherent in their nature."

In spite of our appreciation for that gentleman's ideas in general, such a statement gives us but slight reassurance. Mankind is not a sufficiently logical creature to make us confident of that evolution. We better feel the force of our philosopher's other prognostication: "The time will come when every club for the propagation of nakedness will have its chaplain. In fact Dean Inge has already expressed himself entirely in favour of our taking off our clothes."

For it is conceivable that nudity should in time come to be freed in American minds from its present shameful connotations; in all probability, once we bring ourselves to think about the matter rationally, it will come to be *fairly* "respectable." Not that it will even then cease to arouse the strongest sort of antagonisms—as it has in Germany in the past and does in France today—but certainly it will in the end be viewed calmly and sanely by all who are intellectually capable of viewing any matter in that fashion.

When that time comes, there will be nudists in America, as

surely as there are in Europe. They may not be organized into *Bunds* and *Ligas;* there may never be a concerted nudist movement in America. But those who come to recognize any of the innumerable benefits ascribed to nudity will not let traditional views on modesty and shame deprive them of those advantages. They will practise it, if not publicly then privately.

Naturally the practice would be easiest, most feasible, for the inhabitants of rural communities. For it is the country that offers both the greatest benefits from nudity and the most opportunities for its practice. Yet probably the urbanite will be the first to adopt it, not only because the rural dweller is as a rule less open to the logic of new and still unconventional ideas, but because his urban cousin will feel more the urge to seek the open air and sun of which his city life so largely deprives him.

Nudity will appeal particularly to the younger people of our huge metropolitan populations, the young fathers and mothers sufficiently modern to hold to the current ideas on health and child education. And were the writers of this book to hazard any sort of a prophecy regarding the course that nudity will take in America, they would foretell the eventual rise of small private clubs and nudist fields in or near the larger cities—"Franklin Clubs" and "Thoreau Associations" and "Whitman Societies," possibly—supported mostly by these younger and more enlightened elements of our urban populations.

Yet before anything of that sort can come to be, these younger city inhabitants will first initiate themselves and their children in their own homes or during infrequent vacations to spots sufficiently remote from habitation. They will learn—especially if they have as well a love of nature—to make the most of every opportunity to go into the country, where, laying aside their clothes for a day or even a few hours, they and their offspring may benefit and enjoy themselves in the open air. Only then will they come to practise nudity in small groups of their most intimate associates.

For if the nudist movement has a future in America, it is to be found in individual conviction and practice—which may or may not in time assume the proportions of a concerted movement—rather than in organized propaganda and wholesale conversions. It will be only as eager and voluntary recruits that Americans will don "the shadowed livery of the burnished sun."

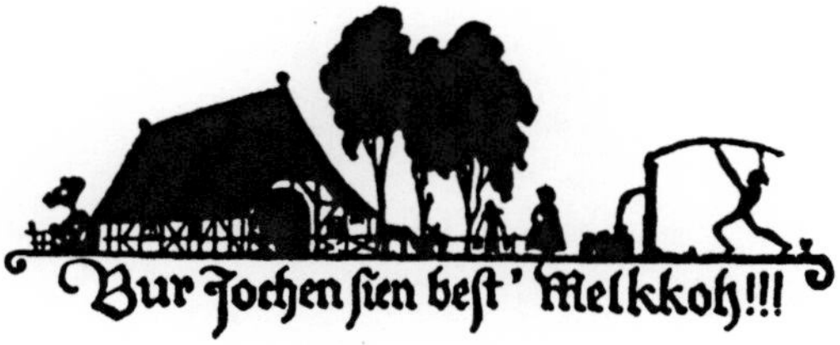
Bur Jochen sien best' Melkkoh!!!

This book is set in Garamond, a modern rendering of the type first cut in the sixteenth century by Claude Garamont (1510–1561.) He was a pupil of Geofroy Tory and is believed to have based his letters on the Venetian models, although he introduced a number of important differences, and it is to him that we owe the letter which we know as Old Style. He gave to his letters a certain elegance and a feeling of movement which won for their creator an immediate reputation and the patronage of the French King, Francis I.

Lightning Source UK Ltd.
Milton Keynes UK
30 August 2009

143183UK00001B/80/A

9 781846 641398